COMING HOME TO YOUR BODY

Other books by Carmen Renee Berry

When Helping You is Hurting Me: Escaping the Messiah Trap
(Harper & Row, 1988)

Loving Yourself as Your Neighbor
A Recovery Guide for Christians Escaping Burnout & Codependency
(with Mark Lloyd Taylor)
(Harper & Row, 1990)

How to Escape the Messiah Trap: A Workbook
(HarperSanFrancisco, 1991)

Are You Having Fun Yet?
How to Bring the Art of Play Into Your Recovery
(Thomas Nelson, 1992)

Is Your Body Trying to Tell You Something?
How Massage and Body Work Can Help You Understand
Why You Feel the Way You Do
(Previously titled *Your Body Never Lies*)
(PageMill Press, 1993)

girlfriends: Invisible Bonds, Enduring Ties
(with Tamara Traeder)
(Wildcat Canyon Press, 1995)

Who's To Blame?
Escape the Victim Trap & Gain Personal Power in Your
Relationships
(with Mark W. Baker)
(Piñon Press, 1996)

The girlfriends Keepsake Book: The Story of Our Friendship
(with Tamara Traeder)
(Wildcat Canyon Press, 1996)

COMING HOME TO YOUR BODY

365 Simple Ways to Nourish Yourself Inside and Out

CARMEN RENEE BERRY

Poetry by Juanita Ryan

PAGEMILL PRESS
A Division of Circulus Publishing Group, Inc.
Berkeley, California

Publisher: Tamara C. Traeder
Editorial Director: Roy M. Carlisle
Copyeditor: Priscilla Stuckey
Cover and Interior Design: Gordon Chun Design
Typesetting: Holly A. Taines, Circulus Publishing Group, Inc.
Typographic Specifications: Body text set in Adobe Garamond 11/14.5,
daily title in 18-point Eva Antiqua Light.
Printed in the United States of America

Library of Congress Cataloging-in-Publication Data
Berry, Carmen Renee.
    Coming home to your body: 365 simple ways to nourish yourself inside
and out / Carmen Renee Berry.
        p. cm.
    Includes index.
    ISBN 1-879290-07-3 (pbk.)
    1. Women—Health and hygiene. 2. Self-care, Health. 3. Women—
Mental health. 4. Stress management. 5. Mind and body.
    I. Title.
    RA778.B524   1996
    613—dc20   96-18632   CIP

Distributed to the trade by Publishers Group West
10 9 8 7 6 5 4 3 2

Dedication

To Carolyn J. Braddock

Who recognized that I was wandering
and guided me back home.

Acknowledgments

My favorite part of writing this book is the opportunity to thank the wonderful people who have contributed to its birth. My first thanks must go to my body work clients, the many adventurous women who invite me to join them in the process of deeper self-knowledge. Not only am I privileged to participate in their exploration, but they have allowed me to share some of their stories of hope and healing with you.

Secondly, I want to thank the courageous and cantankerous women in my Making Peace with Your Body support groups. My life is fuller due to the honest, humorous, and healing experiences we've shared together. Thank you Kitty, Heidi, Karen, Kim, Arleen, Pat, Katie, Carolyn, Laura, and Marianne.

A special thanks is due to those people who have helped to keep my personal life on an even keel during this writing process: to Marianne Croonquist for keeping my home clean (and resisting the urge to vacuum my office when manuscript pages were everywhere); to Lynn Barrington for insisting that I practice what I preach regarding self-care; to Rene Chansler for understanding why I spent so many weekends at the word processor and for insisting that I take time off for a movie every now and then; to Pat Luehrs for consistently offering a unique insight into our many discussions; to Gail Walker with whom I share a love for spas and massage; to Dan Psaute who prays for me daily; to Joel Miller for sharing weekends away in Santa Barbara with me; and to Bob Parsons and Cathy Smith for always, always, always being there for me. I also want to thank all my friends and colleagues at Christian Recovery International who, through the ups and downs, continue to root for the completion of this manuscript.

Among my friends are those who helped me directly with the book's content, including Irene Flores who gave generously of her knowledge about skin care and nutrition, Susan Latta who taught me more about embodied wisdom than she'll ever know, Constance Lillas whose theoretical model regarding states of attention and the body serve as a foundation for my body work, Juanita Ryan whose poetry captured not only her personal journey but mine as well, and my massage therapists—Mandy Steven, Claudette Renner, Charles Swan, Karen Grusznynski, and Steve Jones—whose healing touch taught me about my own body's wisdom.

I don't know whether to jump up and down with elation or fall on my face in sheer gratitude to express how I feel about the fabulous team at Circulus Publishing Group. Roy M. Carlisle, who has served as editor for every book I've written, had a vision for this book long before the first word was typed. Julienne Bennett's enthusiasm for the project seems to know no bounds and kept me motivated. Tamara Traeder's brilliant wit got me laughing so hard that I barely noticed she was asking me to do yet another rewrite. This woman is magnificent. Last, but in no way least, is Holly A. Taines who hung in to the very end with emotional support and an invaluable eye for detail. Thank you!

Author's Note

1. Please note that the author is not a medical practitioner and this book is in no way intended to serve as a substitute for professional medical advice or as a comprehensive guide to health care. This book contains suggestions for exercises and certain food recipes, and any person who is considering making a change to his or her diet, exercise pattern, or lifestyle should first consult with a physician. This applies especially to anyone with a medical condition or suspected medical condition, or who is restricted in their movement, taking medication or on a special diet. Further, the exercises and self-massage techniques included in this book are meant to be pleasurable and relaxing. If, at any time, pain or discomfort is felt while practicing them, one should stop immediately and consult a medical practitioner before trying them again.

2. To preserve my clients' anonymity I have disguised and changed identifiable characteristics whenever possible. Most of the examples in this book are composite portraits, that is, generalized descriptions that draw related points from several different clients' stories. In addition to protecting confidentiality more effectively, composites allow for more broadly applicable examples.

3. The author relied on various sources of material for this book which are listed in the Suggestions for Further Reading list found on pages 399 and 400. Any quotations which are not immediately identified in the text can be found in these books, or in various quote books which provide inspiration. These books include *The Quotable Woman* (Philadelphia, PA: Running Press, 1991), *The New Quotable Woman: The Definitive Treasury of Notable Words by Women from Eve to the Present*, compiled and edited by Elaine Partnow

(New York: Penguin Books, 1992), and *Peter's Quotations: Ideas for Our Time*, by Dr. Laurence J. Peter (New York: Bantam Books, 1977). The author gratefully acknowledges the wisdom and knowledge offered in these volumes.

4. With grateful acknowledgment, biblical quotations are taken from:

The *New Revised Standard Version* (NRSV) published by the Division of Christian Education of the National Council of the Churches of Christ in the U.S.A. (1989).

The *New American Standard Bible* (NASB) published by The Lockman Foundation (1973).

JANUARY

THE WIND

For a very long time
I tried to hold still.
I contained myself.
Frozen stiff. Unmoving.

Then one day a warm wind
spun itself around me
defrosting me
and throwing me off balance.

I was moving.
Stumbling, turning,
and with each changing motion
came new freedom and surprise.

I am no stone statue.
I am alive!

Love the Body You Have

The body is a sacred garment.
—MARTHA GRAHAM, *Blood Memory* (1991)

Looking down at her body, my client said, "I can't accept my body the way it is. Look at me." Her eyes met mine. "I'm overweight and I need to change. If I accept myself, then it's like giving up. I need to reject my body if I'm ever going to lose this weight."

My client voiced what so many women feel: We *should* hate our bodies. If we accept our bodies, the idea goes, we'll stay the way we are. Rejecting our bodies will motivate us to change our bodies, thereby making ourselves acceptable.

This is a lie. So why do women believe it? Perhaps a better question is: Why *wouldn't* we believe it? Look around us. We are told many times a day that our bodies are not good enough. Through print and TV ads we're informed that our bodies emit various offensive odors. Supermodels let us know that our hair isn't shiny enough, our legs aren't thin enough, our breasts aren't large enough, and our hands aren't smooth enough. The answer, of course, is to buy products that will remedy our bodies' deficiencies. The information we're given about our bodies is not intended to give us accurate information about who we are as women, rather it is intended to create a sense of unrest, dissatisfaction, and shame so we'll purchase the advertised wares.

Without realizing it, we have accepted the unspoken message of advertising: If you don't like yourself, you will make better choices. If you don't like your body odor, you'll buy brand X deodorant. If you're embarrassed by your size, you'll buy a new exercise machine or sign up for the newest diet program. If you're dissatisfied with the appearance of your skin, you'll get an expensive jar of night cream. The list can go on and on. If you want a better life, if you want to be attractive, and ultimately if you want to be loved, start by disliking your body.

This message is especially damaging to us when we are ill, have been in accidents, or are aging. We're yoked with the impossible task of staying forever young, seeing any physical limitation as a betrayal by our bodies. Our bodies are our enemies, and pain is the weapon used against us. In a misguided attempt to be healthy, we battle against ourselves, growing angrier, wishing to cut ourselves off from our bodies altogether.

Hostility toward your body is helpful to companies selling products, but not to you. I've never known any woman who made better choices about her body motivated by self-loathing. I've watched women who are ashamed of their bodies lose weight only to gain it all back again. Some of my clients retard healing from illness or car accidents by blaming their bodies for the pain. My personal favorite is overtaxing my body to accomplish professional goals and then blaming my body when I get sick.

We make better choices about our bodies the more we value our bodies. As a writer, I buy paper by the case. If a blank piece of paper is torn, I don't care since I've got more. I toss it in the recycling bin. However, the pages upon which I've printed a manuscript are valuable to me, so I set them in a safe place. I value those pages, so I treat them well and protect them.

Similarly, the more we love our bodies, the more likely we are to cultivate positive health habits: eat more nutritious meals, exercise regularly, treat ourselves kindly through an illness, listen to our bodies' wisdom in the healing process. Accepting your body, right now, with all your real and socially fabricated limitations, is the foundation for making better choices for yourself. Come home to your body. Your body is on your side and always has been.

Keep a Body Journal

Suddenly many movements are going on within me, many things are happening, there is an almost unbearable sense of sprouting, of bursting encasements, of moving kernels, expanding flesh.
—MERIDEL LE SUEUR, *Salute to Spring* (1940)

I invite you to join me in an adventure that begins by rejecting traditional notions of the body as an "it," your possession, a beast to be tamed and mastered. Instead, create a new relationship with your body, allowing yourself to be led, taught, wooed, and embraced.

I am the student, my body the teacher as I endeavor to understand more about myself in ways that are not easily described. Sometimes I see myself as a spy trying to crack a secret code. I long to understand the language of my body.

Become the student, the spy, searcher of priceless knowledge and treasure. Today, tune in to your breath. How are you breathing right now? Deeply? Shallowly? Are you breathing at all? Many of my clients forget to breathe for long periods of time. Next, identify the emotion your breath is expressing, such as relaxation, anxiety, or irritation. What can you learn from your breathing pattern?

If you don't keep a body journal, this is the ideal time to start one. Get a notebook with unlined sheets of paper or a bound book with empty pages. Throughout the year, I'll ask you to use your journal to keep track of the images, sensations, insights, feelings, and messages you receive from your body. Follow your body's lead, and you'll be led back home.

Celebrate Your Back with TLC

The vicious cycle clicks in: you are too busy to nurture yourself, but without self-nurturing your life threatens to become one monotonous and stressful day after another.
—JENNIFER LOUDEN, *The Woman's Comfort Book* (1992)

I walked my last massage client to the door, noticing an aching in my lower back. I had gotten a bit lazy and stood incorrectly during the sessions. Now my lower back ached, my breathing was shallow, and I was emotionally tired. Whenever I put too much stress on my back muscles they let me know they're unhappy with me.

If you experience serious back pain, consult your doctor immediately. But if you know that you've been overdoing it lately, then the pain can serve as a guide to better behavior on your part. You can sit or stand in a more aligned posture, lift less weight and rely more on your legs than your back for strength, or you can avoid activities that put undue stress on your lower back muscles.

When your back muscles are especially sore you can make peace with them by giving them some TLC.

T = Take pressure off your back by resting as much as possible. Often two or three days is required to allow swelling to subside.

L = Let someone massage your back. Be careful not to put strong pressure directly on the muscles that are strained. Rather, massage around the area to increase circulation for relaxation and healing.

C = Commit yourself to stretching and strengthening exercises once you feel well enough to get out of bed. Include your stomach muscles as well as your back muscles in this plan. Often lower back strain can be prevented if your stomach muscles are strong and well conditioned.

Assess Your Stress

Everything in life that we really accept undergoes a change.
—KATHERINE MANSFIELD, *Journal of Katherine Mansfield* (1927)

I instructed one of my massage clients, "Relax your arm." With her eyes closed she responded, "My arm is relaxed."

I smiled. "Open your eyes and take a look for yourself." Her arm was extended straight into the air with her elbow locked. Every muscle in her arm was taut.

She smiled with me. "I guess I don't realize how tense I really am," she breathed as she allowed her arm to relax.

We can't lower the stress in our lives if we haven't faced the fact that we have too much stress. Many of us, like my client, are accustomed to tension in our bodies, unfamiliar with what it would feel like to release it. Each month, I'll ask you to assess your stress so that you can see the progress you are making as the days and weeks go by.

In your body journal, draw an outline of your body. Using colored pens or pencils, color in the areas of your body that are carrying stress right now. You may have a headache, tight neck muscles, or a cramp in your calf. Your stomach may be upset or you may even be forgetting to breathe. Start at your head and work down your entire body, checking in with each part to see if stress has landed there.

If you're like me, you'll discover stress in parts of your body you've never noticed. And noticing is enough for today. Just by accepting the fact that your body is overly stressed, you will let your body know you're paying better attention. That's a good step in the direction of making needed changes.

Share a Meal

A smiling face is half the meal.
—LATVIAN PROVERB

To study the impact of diet on the development of cholesterol, a group of scientists fed several groups of rabbits food that they suspected wasn't good for them (or us). When the scientists looked at the results, they found that the rabbits from all the groups except one did indeed have high cholesterol. This puzzled the scientists because this healthy group of rabbits had eaten the same diet as the unhealthy ones.

They investigated further and found out that the technician who fed this group of rabbits was a kind, nurturing fellow. He didn't just throw the food into the cages. He took time with the rabbits, cuddling them, stroking them, singing to them. Without intending to, this man showed that love can help our bodies metabolize food much better, even food that isn't supposed to be healthy for us. Next time you eat, share a meal with someone who demonstrates love and acceptance. Your food will digest better and you'll be healthier if you do.

Plan a Pap Smear

*As I see it, every day you do one of two things: build health or
produce disease in yourself.*
—ADELLE DAVIS, *Let's Eat Right to Keep Fit* (1954)

I've worked with many women who avoid regular gynecological
exams because of fear or in reaction to abuse in their past. I can
understand. I've never met a woman who likes getting a Pap smear,
whether she's been previously traumatized or not. I'd rather do a
great many things than walk into that doctor's office, so to get myself
there I treat myself to a banana split after the exam.

No matter how awful it feels to you emotionally, getting your
annual exam can literally mean the difference between life and death.
So take your emotional resistance seriously, and do whatever it takes
to get yourself in to the doctor's office on a regular basis for your
Pap smear. Get a girlfriend to go with you. Take yourself shopping
afterward. Ask your spouse or partner to treat you to dinner.

If you've been putting off setting up an appointment, call your
doctor today. If you already have made your appointment, treat
yourself today for taking good care of yourself.

Read Your Body's Story

She seems to have had the ability to stand firmly on the rock of her past while living completely and unregrettably in the present.
—MADELEINE L'ENGLE, *The Summer of the Great-Grandmother* (1974)

Your body tells your story, your entire story. The question is, can you consciously tell that same story from beginning to end, without gaps or confusion?

Researchers have found that women who are able to tell their entire story, even the sad and difficult parts, are much more successful in life than are women who may have suffered less but are confused about their past. Many of the women who come to me for body work have gaps in their memories and are unsure about events in their childhoods. They are working with their bodies to uncover clues, bits of truth that will allow them to piece together the whole story.

Like many women, I hid the truth about my past from myself. I was afraid that I couldn't take it. But, finding out that I was molested by a woman when I was an infant actually freed me to move on with my life. I don't have any more gaps now. I can tell my story from beginning to the present day, and it makes sense.

I encourage you, if you are struggling with unknowns from your childhood, to continue recovering your whole story. No matter how difficult that story may turn out to be, you have survived it. Once you can tell the complete story, your body will be able to relax in the knowledge that the truth is known.

Find the Winter Sun

There seems to be so much more winter than we need this year.
—KATHLEEN NORRIS, *Bread into Roses* (1937)

When I was in graduate school I lived in a magical place in northern Arizona called Oak Creek Canyon. In the summer, the canyon offers welcome shade and green coolness from the hot red heat of Sedona. But in the winter, the days are short and dark, with the sun peeking through only two or three hours before dropping behind the red walls of the canyon. What in the summer had been a comforting haven became in the winter a prison of dark days and claustrophobic nights. A couple of my neighbors became seriously depressed, hardly able to function. None of us knew about the kind of physiological depression that can result from the lack of sunlight, so we didn't know how to help.

If your mood darkens with the winter sky, you may be suffering from a chemical change in your body due to a need for more sunlight. Rather than minimize your depression as "merely emotional," take seriously the physical component to winter depression. Using full-spectrum fluorescent lights can help give you light that is similar to what we receive from the sun. Even though the weather may be cold, get outside as much as possible to maximize your exposure to the sun. Open up the drapes, sit by the window, and take advantage of every opportunity to enjoy the light.

Locate Compassion in Your Body

*With compassion, we see benevolently our own human
condition. . . . We drop prejudice. We withhold judgment.*
—Christina Baldwin, *Life's Companion:
Journal Writing as a Spiritual Quest* (1990)

Late one night a girlfriend called, tearfully describing the
ending of a relationship with her boyfriend of two years. She
didn't have to invite me over to talk. I felt her sadness in my chest
and her disappointment in my shoulders. I wanted to be near her
as she grieved.

Compassion draws us together to ease the pain we would otherwise suffer alone. Like a magnet, we're pulled toward a loved one
with a desire to care, to respond, to make a difference. I often feel
compassion for others through a tingling in the palms of my hands,
prompting me to lay my hand on their backs or to touch their arms
in reassurance. No words are necessary when one body speaks to
another, conveying the message, "I am here and I care."

Where in your body do you feel compassion's pull? Do you feel
a tug from your heart? A twitching in your hands out of a longing
to touch and soothe the pain? A tightness in your calves as they
spring to respond? In your body journal, record your body's way of
expressing this intimate emotion. Then watch to see who is calling
to you for extra care. Respond to the call and actively express your
compassion.

Put Egg on Your Face

I'm tired of all this nonsense about beauty being only skin-deep.
That's deep enough. What do you want, an adorable pancreas?
—JEAN KERR, *The Snake Has All the Lines* (1958)

I love the winter, especially in southern California, because it's the only time of year we have any noticeable weather at all. Even though our cold and rainy days don't compare in severity with the rest of the country's, my skin lets me know that winter is leaving its mark on my body.

Is your skin dried out by the winter cold? You can rejuvenate your face with ingredients already in your kitchen. Separate two eggs and mix the yolks with some olive oil. Smooth on your face, being careful to avoid your eyes, and let absorb. You can leave this mixture on all night or you can dab off the excess with cotton balls. For a special treatment, substitute ginkgo biloba oil (found at a local health food store) for the olive oil. This mixture will add elasticity and facilitate healing for your chapped skin.

Be Assertive, Be Aware

Assertiveness is the ability to exercise one's own rights without denying the rights of others. This builds upon personal awareness, for a woman must first be in touch with what it is she wants or needs in any given situation.
—BAMM IMPACT, in *Not An Easy Target* (1995)

One week I drove an hour east of Pasadena to present a full-day seminar on how to prevent burnout and take care of yourself. The next day, I rose early to drive into Los Angeles to present two back-to-back workshops on how to prevent burnout and take care of yourself. After the workshops, I caught a plane to Monterey where I presented an evening seminar on how to prevent burnout and take care of yourself. The next morning, I flew to Seattle in time to give a keynote address on, you guessed it, how to prevent burnout and take care of yourself. My back ached, my throat hurt, my feet throbbed. Anyone besides my body see a problem here?

I have learned to be an assertive caregiver. I am fierce when fighting for someone I love or something I believe in. But when it comes to advocating for myself, I haven't been that adept. In fact, I still find it hard to know what I need or want.

My body, however, is very aware of my needs. My stomach rumbles when I need to eat. My eyes droop when I need to sleep. My palms sweat when I need to protect my boundaries. My jaw clenches when I need to express anger.

Take out your body journal. Answer the question, "What does my body tell me I need?" Then use your assertiveness abilities (which most women use for the defense of others) to advocate for yourself. Notice your breathing, posture, and which muscles feel tight.

Show Up for Sex

True love needs the foundation of physical affection.
—DAPHNE ROSE KINGMA, *True Love* (1991)

Not tonight, dear. I have a headache. With this stereotypical response, a woman brushes off her husband's desire for sex. Typically we think that men want more sex and women, who often feel emotionally ignored, want less. I've worked with couples where the roles were reversed. Regardless of gender, couples can fall into an unfortunate pattern of distancing from each other, one wanting to communicate love primarily through physical contact and the other primarily through emotional or verbal interaction. Who is right? Both are.

A complete expression of love requires both bodily and emotional presence. When we pull the physical away from the emotional and spiritual aspects of love, we cut love in half and it dies.

In order to be fully present during lovemaking, both partners must be fully connected to their bodies. If you have trouble staying in your body during intimacy, this may be a signal that additional healing needs to take place between you and your body. I recommend talking with a therapist who works with body issues as well as seeking out a professional body worker who is trained in healing the body-mind split. You owe it to yourself to fully enjoy your sexuality. Do whatever you need to be fully present emotionally, spiritually, and physically.

Drink to Your Health

The best thing to do with water is to use a lot of it.
—PHILIP JOHNSON, *The New Yorker*, July 9, 1966

Did you know that two-thirds of your body is water? Take a look at a piece of dried fruit. That's how we'd all look without water in our bodies. Water makes up our blood and lymph fluid, allowing them to flow throughout our systems carrying nutrients to our tissue and carrying waste away. Your body produces two liters of lymph fluid every day. To produce all that fluid, your body needs some help.

So, drink up! Go for eight eight-ounce glasses of water a day. If that seems boring, then spruce it up by garnishing your water with sprigs of mint or slices of lemon. Pour water into a fancy glass or drink it completely naked for a change of pace. Whatever it takes, drink lots of water. Every cell in your body will thank you for it.

Sink into a Sacred Sleep

*The great lesson from the mystics . . . is that
the sacred is in the ordinary.*
—Abraham Maslow, *Religions, Values, and Peak-Experiences* (1964)

What could possibly be more ordinary and less "sacred" than falling asleep? Everyone does it at an average rate of once a day.

Tonight, turn an ordinary experience into a time of embodied spirituality. After all your chores are completed, take a warm bath or shower, washing away the day's concerns. After gently toweling yourself dry, dress in something you especially like to wear to bed— a luxurious nightgown or a sloppy, soft T-shirt. Light a candle by your bed, cut off all other lights, and sit for a few moments on the side of the bed observing how the candlelight plays off all the walls. Let the candle glow turn your ordinary bedroom into a sanctuary.

Stretch out on the bed and take a deep breath. Let your attention move slowly from your feet to the top of your head, relaxing each part as you go. Once relaxed, read a portion from a book of poetry, scripture, or some other writing that honors the body. Let the encouragement and comfort sink deep into your body until you can feel the spiritual nurturance in your bones. Listen for God's voice. Then blow out the candle and drift into a sound and delicious sleep.

Laugh Away the Blues

Laughter is by definition healthy.
—DORIS LESSING, *The Summer Before the Dark* (1973)

Not too long ago I was feeling depressed. A friend of mine dropped by with a video and, even though I initially protested, she finally talked me into watching it with her. A couple hours later, after laughing continuously through the romantic comedy, my mood had lifted considerably. There's nothing like laughter to alter our physiology, giving us an extra burst of energy and feelings of optimism.

Here is a surefire recipe for curing the blues:

♦ Select one humorous video.

♦ Mix with an evening with the phone off the hook.

♦ Add a large bowl of unsalted popcorn, sprinkled lightly with Parmesan cheese.

♦ Wrap yourself around something soft (such as a lover, dog, cat, or stuffed animal).

♦ And let the mood rise as you laugh to your heart's content.

You'll feel better, your immune system will be strengthened, your digestion will improve, and you'll enjoy better blood circulation. What more could you ask from an evening at home?

Start a New Habit

Human beings have a tendency to gravitate toward repetitive
patterns. Habits or patterns require less energy
and seem to make life simpler.
—CAROL C. WELL, *Right-Brain Sex* (1989)

D id you know that our brains are constructed so that we can "lock in" a habit in about twenty-one days? If you do something new consistently for three weeks, chances are you'll continue this new behavior indefinitely without having to discipline yourself or even pay attention.

What new, positive habit would you like to have in your life at the end of three weeks? Ask your body what changes may be needed to keep yourself healthy, and decide on a new habit you are willing to develop. Here are a few ideas:

♦ Get to bed on time.

♦ Take five minutes each day to stretch out your muscles.

♦ Eat fresh fruit every day.

Get out your calendar and mark three weeks from today so you'll be able to see how your life has changed for the better in such a short time. Ready to start a new habit? Great. Let's go.

Celebrate Your Voice

The voice is a wild thing. It can't be bred in captivity.
—WILLA CATHER, *The Song of the Lark* (1915)

I heard a whisper on the phone line, wondering if this would turn out to be an obscene call. "Carmen? I've lost my voice."

It was my friend, Lynn, a personal career coach who talks on the phone to dozens of songwriters each week. Even though she needed time off, Lynn had pushed herself. Her body spoke loudly through her raspy whisper, making a decision to rest that Lynn couldn't refuse.

Ever hear the phrase "silence is golden?" That may be true for someone wanting to sleep in, but it's not so much fun if you use your voice in your work or you're in the mood to sing but can't due to laryngitis. If your larynx becomes infected or irritated, the natural vibrations required to create your normal speaking and singing voice are disrupted. You may end up with a deep, throaty, "sexy" voice or a high-pitched, intermittent, "helium" voice.

If you come down with laryngitis, give your voice time to heal. Avoid talking whenever possible, and drink plenty of warm liquids such as chamomile or ginger tea. And, of course, don't smoke or hang out in smoke-filled rooms. If it continues, see a doctor.

Instead of talking out loud, silently ask, "What does this mean?" Maybe you felt a cold coming on but didn't stop at the first sign to take care of yourself. Perhaps you need to "speak your truth" but have been unwilling to take the risk. Did you spend time with someone who smokes, allowing second-hand smoke to inflame your throat and lungs? Since you won't be talking much, you'll have plenty of time to listen for the answer.

Remember Who You Are

In violence, we forget who we are.
—MARY MCCARTHY, *On the Contrary* (1961)

I asked a client, "Does this hurt?" as I pressed on a particularly tight knot in her leg.

"No, why should it?" she asked. "It's a bone."

It wasn't a bone but rather a part of her muscle that was so tight it felt numb. Many of my clients have "numb knots," through which no sensation, pain, and pleasure, are felt. Often these clients are survivors of some kind of physical, emotional, or sexual violence.

Violence is, first and foremost, a crime against the body. Our bodies are used as weapons against us, as pain is inflicted via our physical beings. If we are unable to avoid the slaps, hits, or shoves perpetrated on us, we may protect ourselves by numbing ourselves to the pain itself. Some clients describe floating above their bodies and watching themselves endure painful moments. Others seem to "zone out" and remember little to nothing about an abusive experience. Still others no longer respond to physical sensations of pain or pleasure, wearing their bodies like overcoats.

We cannot know ourselves fully or accurately if we are floating, zoning, or numbing. We must be grounded, alert, and alive to the range of sensation. Take a stand against violence not by pulling away from your body but by drawing all the closer. You might walk on the carpet in bare feet, feeling yourself solid, supported by the earth. Or, you may take several deep breaths, imagining the oxygen flowing all the way to your toes. One of my favorites is to lie on the floor and stretch each part of my body, feeling fully embodied.

Remember who you are. If you've forgotten, your body is ready to tell you.

Get a Body Buddy

Friendship always benefits . . .
—SENECA, in ALEXANDRA STODDARD, *Daring To Be Yourself* (1990)

Several years back I was invited to spend the day with a couple of male friends and a woman they knew named Susan. She and I hit it off immediately, chatting the whole day about massage and body work. Within a few weeks, we set up a women's support group that we nicknamed The Body Group, and for the next three years, we met regularly to talk about what we were learning about ourselves from our bodies.

Talking with other women who are exploring the mysteries of the body is a priceless gift. Today, pick up the phone and call a woman you know is able to nurture you as well as receive your love. Ask her if she'd like to be your "body buddy," a friend who travels with you as you both make peace with your body. You may want to meet on a regular basis to discuss what you both are learning about your bodies. From time to time, you may want to share your body journals with each other. What is shared between you is held in confidence, making it safe to discuss your triumphs and difficulties openly.

Enjoy your body buddy as soon as possible by arranging to share a meal together. Expect at least half of the nourishment to come from the food and half from her love for you.

Move Like a Youngster

After thirty, a body has a mind of its own.
—BETTE MIDLER, in *Reader's Digest* (1982)

Are you in the same argument with your body that I am with mine? I want everything to work the same way it did when I was nineteen. Needless to say, this is one argument I'm definitely losing.

Medical research tells us that aging picks up speed around the age of thirty. Dr. James Liles, a professor at the University of Tennessee, says a person can noticeably slow down the aging process by exercising three times a week for thirty minutes to an hour. Otherwise, the capacity of our hearts, respiratory organs, kidneys, and a number of other vital functions are thought to decrease by about one percent a year after thirty.

So, if you aren't committed to a regular exercise regime, today's the day to start. And if you're already a regular exerciser, then congrats to you! You're younger than you think.

Stop

A spiritual retreat is medicine for soul starvation.
—DAVID COOPER, *Silence, Simplicity, and Solitude* (1992)

I was angry at God, again, for the confusion raging through my brain and the disappointment searing my heart. "Why do you seem so far away?" I fumed. "Why don't I have a sense of direction?" Racing from appointment to appointment, I muttered my rage at God with my heart pounding and my teeth clenched. How could I have expected to hear the voice of wisdom with my ears full of my own interior talk and my body stressed and unreceptive?

Imagine what can happen when I stop. When I rest in a sense of trust. When I cease my incessant chatter and finally listen. Then I hear the music of my soul, the truth of nature, the insight available only to those who let their bodies become a conduit for spiritual understanding.

Join me, today, in the spiritual discipline of listening, not simply with your ears but with your entire, quieted body. Lie down in a comfortable position and take several deep breaths. Let go of everything that keeps you from communing with God—your anger, your unbelief, or your anxiety. Release these spiritual barriers from your mind and your body. Notice how your muscles relax, your breathing deepens, and the lines on your face smooth out.

Listen to the pounding of your heart. Notice the rhythm of your breath. Feel the bottoms of your feet, the texture of your clothing against your skin, and the temperature in the room. Ask God to join you in this quiet moment, and to speak to you.

Bathe in Japan

Water is the great purifier of life.
But there is more than one way to take a bath!
—JENNIFER LOUDEN, *The Woman's Comfort Book* (1992)

Stand by the window and imagine Mount Fuji in the distance. Beginning your purification ritual, you boil water and allow green tea to steep. Moving to your bedroom, you slip into a beautiful silk kimono. The softness of the fabric caresses your skin. Pausing, you admire the delicate design and intriguing colors of the kimono. Turning on your tape player, Japanese music soothes you. The incense is lit, filling the room with an aroma of peaceful meditation. You sit, back straight and eyes closed. One breath, another breath, you relax. You travel down, deep, into the center of your soul. For several minutes, you commune with yourself and God.

Once centered, you move to the bath. The hot water streams into the tub as bath oil is poured into the stirring water. Steam fills the room with fragrance. You tape travel posters to the walls of the bathroom. Japanese splendor surrounds you—green mountains rising above the mist, rice fields spreading out for miles, tranquil and carefully manicured gardens offering places of refuge and rest.

Ahh . . . you sink into the warmth of the bath and the nurturing view of Asian countryside. You meditate, imagining yourself in each scene, perhaps as a Japanese monk or a noble samurai or a European explorer seeing the Asian mysteries for the first time.

It's time to return from Japan. But before you leave, you pause, savor the tea, breathe in the fragrance, relax in the liquid nurturance, and feel grateful for the joys of your senses.

Rate Your Self-Acceptance

*There's a period of life when we swallow a knowledge of ourselves
and it becomes either good or sour inside.*
—PEARL BAILEY, *The Raw Pearl* (1968)

Write in the numbers indicating how often, if ever, the statements are true. Modify those statements that don't apply to you. 1—Never, 2—Sometimes, 3—Always.

___I have a sense of my entire body.

___I rarely fall, trip, or bump into people or things.

___On the whole, I am happy with the way my body looks.

___I live in my body, rarely splitting off or numbing my feelings.

___I pay attention to the messages my body sends me.

___I laugh easily and often.

___I easily and happily accept compliments.

___I enjoy giving and receiving hugs.

___I feel good about the direction my life is taking.

___I protect myself from hurtful criticism.

___I stand firmly and comfortably on both of my feet.

___I breathe regularly and deeply.

___My "self-talk" is positive and encouraging.

___I hold my head up high and my shoulders back.

___I regularly receive massage to increase my self-esteem.

Scoring Evaluation

37-45   Great! You enjoy a positive relationship with your body.
26-36   Watch out. Your body deserves more respect.
0-25   Body alert! Your relationship with your body needs repair.

Celebrate Your Mind

The mind can no longer be thought of as being confined to the brain or to the intellect; it exists in every cell of our bodies.
—CHRISTIANE NORTHRUP, M.D., *Women's Bodies, Women's Wisdom* (1994)

When I took biology in high school and college, I was taught that the nerves carried information from different parts of the body to the brain and vice versa. It was believed that chemical messengers called neuropeptides, which convey emotions and thoughts, traveled solely in the brain and along the nerves. But recent research has discovered that receptors for these messengers are located all over the body, including in our immune systems, endocrine systems and organs.

Think about how this information changes the way we view our bodies. Dr. Northrup writes, "Our entire body feels and expresses emotion—all parts of us 'think' and 'feel.'" Our emotions and thoughts emerge, not solely from the brain, but directly from all parts of our bodies—from muscles, bladder, uterus, lungs, every part of us. We can no longer scientifically justify the mind-body split that Westerners have believed in for centuries. There is no division. We are, indeed, whole.

So feel with your pancreas, think with your toes, emote through your breasts, and ponder truth with your bowels. Celebrate the unity of your body and mind today.

Be Hard to Follow

Misfortune had made Lily supple instead of hardening her, and a
pliable substance is less easy to break than a stiff one.
—EDITH WHARTON, *The House of Mirth* (1905)

Protecting ourselves from unscrupulous people requires a higher level of attention and flexibility than needed in the past. A growing pattern of assault, at least in the city in which I live, includes follow-home robberies and carjackings. Thieves may spot you at the mall, a restaurant, or other public place and watch you drive away. Experts tell us that usually carjackers work in pairs so that they can follow you home, with one person jumping from their vehicle to assault you, leaving the second person free to drive their car away from the scene of the crime.

The best protection against being followed home is to be aware of your surroundings. If you suspect that you're being followed, try this simple test described by Craig Fox Huber and Don Paul in *Secure from Crime*. Turn right four times. It's possible that the car behind you happens to be turning right once or twice. Maybe even three times. But if the car follows you in a complete circle, the car is following you. Don't go home but drive straight to the nearest police station or a busy gas station or restaurant. Report the car to the police, even though, by this time, the car is most likely hightailing it to the other side of town looking for a less alert target.

Grow Large on Love

*Loneliness and the feeling of being unwanted
is the most terrible poverty.*
—MOTHER TERESA, in *Time magazine* (1975)

My client told me, "Had it not been for my children, their love and my love for them, I would never have gotten out of bed in the morning. In fact, I may never have gotten out of bed again but given up and died."

Loneliness is not merely a matter of the metaphorical heart. Feeling unloved and adrift, beyond the reach of a caressing touch or listening ear, can permeate our bodies on a cellular level. Infants who are well fed will waste away and even die if their hunger for affection is not satisfied. The best medical care proves impotent if we've lost the will to live.

Our bodies grow lean and sickly without the experience of *being with* others. Some bodies show their emotional starvation through thin limbs and sagging skin. Others hide their spiritual poverty under layers of cellulite. But beneath the padding is a person dying from love hunger.

Take a good look at yourself, your body, and your soul. Are you withering away from a diet of loneliness or growing large and healthy on the nourishment of love? Nourish yourself with a short phone conversation with your body buddy. Open yourself to the feast and reclaim, not only your reason, but your capacity to live.

Rest a Fever

Everyone who is born holds dual citizenship, in the
kingdom of the well and in the kingdom of the sick.
—SUSAN SONTAG, *Illness as Metaphor* (1978)

She sat on the couch with red, watery eyes, shoulders slumped
and shivering slightly. Her voice had a nasal twang as she said,
"I think I'm coming down with the flu, but since I'd already made
the appointment, I thought I should come."

Every so often, sick but responsible souls with stuffed noses,
aching joints, and coughing lungs stagger toward my massage table.
Why? Because they feel obligated to keep their appointments. And
each time I send them home *sans* massage. I'm impressed by these
women's responsibility. The problem is that they feel responsible
to meet an expectation they imagine I have, and they overlook their
true responsibility to their own bodies. My instructions to go home
and rest are met with a combination of surprise and relief—surprise
that I would honor their bodies in such a demonstrable way and
relief because that's what they've been secretly wanting to do all
day.

If you're sick, especially if you have a fever, contact your doctor,
stay in bed, and drink plenty of clear fluids. A massage can help
you feel better when you're healthy, but it can make you feel worse
if you have a cold or flu. The lymph system may be overstimulated,
causing your symptoms to worsen.

Live up to your body's expectations. Resist the urge to over-
medicate yourself with over-the-counter remedies and to drag
yourself to work. Rest, drink lots of clear fluids, and give your body
a chance to heal. Your body is really good at healing if you cooperate
with the process.

Mail Yourself a Good Idea

Nothing dies harder than a bad idea.
—JULIA CAMERON, *The Artist's Way* (1992)

In the land of Greece, some four hundred years before the birth of Christ, philosophers like Plato and Socrates decided that there was a division between the body and the spirit and that the body was bad and the spirit was good. In fact, Plato believed that the body was the prison of the soul, which would be released only through death.

Now that's a bad idea.

And here we are, centuries later, suffering the impact of this destructive concept. I say it's high time to put an end to this offensive and inaccurate perspective. How about a burial ritual to communicate to your body and your unconscious that you mean business?

Invite a couple friends, if you'd like, and gather around a fireplace or some other safe container for burning. Write on pieces of paper some of the "bad" ideas you've had about your body. One by one, burn these ideas and let the smoke rise to release their hold on your heart and mind. After all your bad ideas have been burned, write down new "good" ideas on a piece of paper. List all the things you like about yourself—your gorgeous nails, the color of your eyes, the slope of your shoulders, the tingly way you sneeze, the softness of the skin on the bottom of your feet. Let yourself be positive about yourself. Put the paper in an envelope, address it to yourself and stamp it. Drop it in the mail in the next day or so. Soon you'll receive a letter full of good ideas about your body. What a great gift!

Enjoy the Complexities

*Who would ever think that so much can go on
in the soul of a young girl?*
—ANNE FRANK, *Diary of a Young Girl* (1952)

In high school I had a girlfriend who was highly intelligent and easily bored. I once caught her watching TV, talking on the phone, scanning a novel, and doing her geometry homework—all at the same time. (The infuriating part was that she pulled straight A's in geometry!)

Few of us can consciously master more than a couple of tasks simultaneously. Our bodies, however, are engaged in a myriad of tasks. At this very moment, you are breathing, digesting, metabolizing, eliminating, purifying, pulsing, signaling, restoring, and healing yourself. It's easy to take such a marvel for granted.

Pull out your body journal and make a list of all the activities your body is engaged in at this moment. Include in your list the many things going on inside of you, that require no conscious effort whatsoever to perform. Also notice what your body is doing on a more observable level, such as sitting upright, holding a pen in your hand, chewing gum, looking at the page in your journal, or listening to music playing in the background.

After your list is complete, allow yourself to feel the gratitude warranted. Your body is truly awesome. You are awesome.

Be Yourself

If a woman discovers her own style she will automatically find
creative outlets through which to express herself. . . . Personal style
and self-confidence go hand in hand.
—ALEXANDRA STODDARD, *Daring to Be Yourself* (1990)

Sitting by the restaurant window waiting for a friend, I watched people walk by. Most of the people passed in a blur until a particular woman caught my eye. She didn't call overt attention to herself. She didn't need to, because it was clear that she was perfectly content with herself just the way she was.

Her shoulders were back, resting comfortably on a confident back. The outfit she wore was simple yet striking, with muted colors that drew attention to her easy smile and happy eyes. She had taken time to braid her hair in a novel, flattering pattern that gave me the impression she enjoyed creatively expressing herself through her appearance. As she gracefully disappeared into the crowd, I felt a longing inside myself to know her, to know her magic, her confidence, her calm.

Take time today and go to a public place like a mall, an airport, or a museum—somewhere you can sit and watch people go by. Look for women who appear, to you, to have a high regard for their bodies. Observe how they walk, smile, hold their heads, move their hands, stand on their feet. Notice how different they may be from each other, as no one way to express oneself is "right." When you are ready, take a walk sporting your own special style of confidence. Let your body express how wonderful you feel you are.

Celebrate the Body You Have

How do you accept your body—especially if you've been at war with
it for years? Walk the walk of the Beautiful People. Buy the
fashionable clothes. Wear the forbidden bathing suit. . . .
Accept the dates. Dance. Sing!
—STEVEN C. STRAUSS, M.D., AND GAIL NORTH

Rejecting our bodies results in rejecting the present and all the
opportunities available to us now. We may say to ourselves:

♦ I can't go to the party. I'm too fat and I don't have anything to
wear.

♦ If I were beautiful like she is, I could be successful too.

♦ I'd love to take up skiing, but I've got no energy.

♦ I could never go out dancing. I move like an orangutan.

Those of us who dislike our bodies are always waiting—until we
get thinner, until we feel better, until we change our bodies in some
way that makes us worthy to live in the present. The problem is,
our bodies are never thin, shapely, strong, or something enough, so
we don't get into the game.

Why wait? Live in the present now by loving the body you have.
Love the body you have by saying yes to the next opportunity that
presents itself to you. Go for it!

FEBRUARY

FALLING IN LOVE

I am falling
in love
with life.
This miracle
of grace
came none too soon.

Perhaps it is
that I am
coming to life.
Stirrings deep within.
Awakenings of energy
and hope.

In this harsh
desert landscape
of endless
despair,
a small
wild rose
is blooming.

Be Alert!

*It is not easy to find happiness in ourselves
and it is not possible to find it elsewhere.*
—AGNES REPPLIER (1855-1950)

Even though I've been involved with body work since 1985, there's so much more to learn that the journey remains exciting. While recently working on a book project with a dear friend and colleague, Dr. Constance Lillas, I became acquainted with research about the six states of consciousness, information that has revolutionized how I relate to my body.

The six states are, starting from the bottom: deep sleep, light sleep, drowsy, alert, agitated, and flooded. While the sleep states are self-explanatory, the top three should be explored. When we're in the alert state, we're the happiest we can be. Our food is digesting well, the heart rate is normal, and breathing is deep and regular with blood nurturing our organs. In this state, we have access to any emotion, especially the enjoyable ones. We're calm enough to perceive all the wonderful things going on around us.

Let's say something annoys or frightens us. Our bodies move into the agitated state, and a lot changes rapidly. First, hormones flood our bloodstreams, most notably adrenaline, which gives us extra energy to deal with the threat. We stop digesting food and actually start digesting our own tissue! Breathing is shallow, with heart pounding. Along with these physiological changes, our emotions and intellectual capacities are limited. The more agitated we become, the more we lose the ability to feel positive feelings, and to process thoughts calmly and thoroughly.

As anxiety grows, we can move into the flooded state. Feelings narrow and intensify. For example, anger becomes rage, fear becomes terror, sadness becomes despair. This might occur if we're in a car accident, awakened in the night by an earthquake, yelled at by someone we fear, or reliving a terrible past experience. In this state, the body is prepared to fight or run for survival with adrenaline pumping at maximum level. Normal physiological functioning is stopped so that the emergency can be handled.

Now, why is all this so interesting to me? I realized that I have spent the bulk of my life living in the agitated or flooded states, not in the alert state where I belong. Life can be very stressful, and the more disconnected or at war I've been with my body, the more I've missed important warnings my body was sending. Adrenaline pounded in my veins, and I thought that rush was normal, the way we're supposed to live our lives. But it isn't. In fact, living in the agitated or flooded states will do serious damage to our bodies and can even shorten our lives.

I'm not the only one living life in agitation. Some of my clients grew up in families that were chaotic, cold, or intrusive. Consequently, most weren't taught to calm themselves so that they could be fully alert to their surroundings. As children, they were surviving. Now, as adults, they're learning what they needed to learn as children—how to accurately understand the messages their bodies give and how to cooperate with this embodied wisdom.

Ask yourself what states you experience daily. Do you spend most of the day in an alert state, free to enjoy those in your life, or are you agitated or even overwhelmed much of the time? If you don't know, check out your heart rate, your breath, the tension in your muscles, and the color of your skin. As you learn to read your body more accurately, you'll find your body continuously gives you valuable information about how you are coping—alerting you to take care of yourself.

Insist on Safe Sex

*What seems to be essential to really great sex is not the state of love
but the state of feeling loved. Feeling loved is synonymous
with feeling safe.*
—CAROL C. WELL, *Right-Brain Sex* (1989)

Jean, one of my clients, told me, "Until I received body work, I
didn't know I could say 'no' to my husband. Whatever he wanted,
I felt obligated to give, no matter how I felt. I got through by
pretending to be somewhere else."

I often hear variations on this story. They may love their partners
dearly and want a full, rich sex life, but something happens and the
next thing they know, they're planning the grocery list, floating
above their bodies, or simply zoning out. Their bodies go through
the motions of sex, but they aren't present for the experience.

Women may dissociate as a way to protect themselves. If we
don't feel safe, we seldom feel turned on. Sometimes feeling unsafe
around sex reflects abusive experiences from the past. Some women
fear sex, not because they were directly abused, but because they
think their bodies are flawed and fear rejection. A woman can also
fear intimacy if her relationship with her partner is not secure.
Perhaps she feels dominated, used, or invaded, but does not express
these concerns. Instead, she quietly slips away, leaving her body to
perform sexually, unprotected.

Finding yourself disinterested in sex or drifting off during a sexual
encounter is important information for you to examine. Your body
may be telling you about past abuse. Or you may need to address
issues in your current relationship. Make a commitment to your
body that you will not abandon yourself—staying in your body is a
higher priority than staying in bed when you feel unsafe.

Learn from Your Pain

Listen to the pain message and try not to do anything
that aggravates the pain.
—JAMES F. FRIES, M.D., AND DONALD M. VICKERY, M.D.,
Take Care of Yourself (1993)

If, in one of my workshops, I handed large hat pins to the women saying, "We're going to do an exercise—I want you to stick one of these pins deeply into your thigh," I'd hear gasps of horror, and, I guarantee you, no one would stab herself in the leg.

Why not? Well, to state the obvious, sticking oneself in the leg with a hat pin hurts! And yet, many of us do hurtful things to and with our bodies every day. I confess, I've endured stress headaches instead of pacing myself and saying "no" to overworking. And I've gulped down antacids rather than take a few moments to breathe and listen to the message my stomach was sending. I'm pretty good at ignoring yet aggravating the pain in my life.

And I'm not the only one. Here are a few "ignore and aggravate" patterns I have heard. One woman told me she gets so busy she lets her bladder fill up until she thinks she'll pop. Another woman frets about work, tosses and turns in bed, throws her back out, and then is in so much pain the next day she cannot get any work done. Another woman decides that the extra weight is coming off *now*, religiously attends aerobics classes no matter how much it hurts, and ends up discussing knee surgery.

Sticking a pin in your thigh doesn't sound so odd any more, does it? It's about as reasonable as ignoring your body's guidance while adamantly engaging in self-damaging activities. Hat pin, anyone?

Depend on Dependability

*Replace a habit with a habit. . . . [T]hink well of yourself while you
build trust in the higher order of life—an order that provides an
assurance of dependability.*
—JUDY LYN, *The Sun Always Rises* (1990)

My shelves are full of books defending or refuting the existence of God from an intellectual basis. For years I thought that I would find spiritual assurance somewhere in those pages so I read every book I could. Each time I thought I'd found a line of reasoning that was certain, I'd find another writer who eloquently undermined my confidence. By pursuing spirituality solely in my mind, my thoughts and fears swirled around in my brain like the spinning blades atop a helicopter, lifting me further away from the stability of earth. I lost contact with the predictable rhythms of nature, available to me through my senses. I could not reason my way to spiritual wisdom and comfort.

I'm replacing this spiritually destructive habit with one that practices spirituality rooted in the earth and in God's expression of love through nature. I take comfort in the ebb and flow of life, expressed through the regularity of the ocean's tides and the fact that rebirth always follows the harshest winters.

Replace your disempowering habit with one of confidence, self-love and body love. Start by meditating on the world your senses show you is predictable and trustworthy. Reflect on the fact that day always follows night, gravity always keeps you connected to the earth, and birds always sing after a storm. In a society of over-whelming change, let your senses connect you to a predictable reality based in the comforting and consistent character of God.

Mold Your Body with Kindness

*[L]ike clay, we either keep ourselves moist and malleable or we are
drying and hardening. We must do one or the other . . .*
—DEANE JUHAN, *Job's Body* (1987)

With a tingle of anticipation, I clicked on the exercise video
ready to remold my flabby thighs into rock-hard pillars.
The contrast between my shape and those of the young, slim lovelies
on the tape motivated me to exercise long after my body signaled
me to stop. After forty-five minutes, I watched the remainder of
the video in a exhausted heap on the floor. When I reached for the
remote, my hip muscles had contracted so that I could not stand
erect. I didn't move without pain for the next three days.

As I learned the hard way, we need to mold our bodies with
kindness, not overuse. If we treat our bodies like machines to be
controlled, forcing our muscles beyond their endurance, we can
become old before our time. If, however, we mold ourselves gently,
our muscles grow in strength and elasticity.

By yourself, or with friends, work with clay and see how easy it is
to change its shape. Imagine that your body is like this clay. We
have a great deal of influence over what shape our bodies will take
through the care we give ourselves. Notice as you work the clay
that, without proper moisture, the clay dries out. Our bodies are
similar, needing plenty of water for the body and refreshing love
for the soul.

Mold the clay into a representation of how you view your body.
You can create an actual model of your body or a symbolic representation. After you have finished, write in your journal any insights
or feelings you had during the process. If you are doing this exercise
in a group, share with the other women as you feel comfortable.

Apologize to Your Body

I had to face the facts, I was pear-shaped.
I was a bit depressed because I hate pears.
—CHARLOTTE BINGHAM, *Coronet Among the Weeds* (1963)

I've yet to meet a woman who says, "I just love my body! Don't you think it's grand?"

Nope, we all seem to have at least one thing we find unacceptable if not outright embarrassing or even horrifying. One of my least favorite parts of my body is my nose. All through my adolescence, I stared at my nose in the mirror wishing I could have it changed.

A few years ago, a friend of mine got her nose altered, and through black eyes and bandages, she told me, "I just want a nose like yours." I wish I had a video of the expression on my face, because I was stunned. I was sure that everyone on the planet felt sorry for me because of my nose. It never occurred to me that someone might actually want her nose to be shaped like mine.

Take some time and think about a part of your body you don't especially like. Thank that part of yourself for remaining a part of your body in spite of your ungrateful attitude. And then do something nice for your body part today. That part of you has had to put up with a lot of criticism. It's time to apologize.

Celebrate Your Joints

*The strength of our human scaffolding is incredible. Bone can
withstand a stress of twenty-four thousand pounds per square inch, or
about four times the stress capability of steel.*
—CARL KOCH AND JOYCE HEIL, *Created in God's Image* (1991)

Not long ago, I massaged too many clients in one day, resulting in swelling around my fingers' joints. As I earn my living with my hands through massage and writing, a decreased capacity in my hands would be life-changing.

Taking care of our joints is crucial for maintaining a life of mobility—for walking, dancing, caressing, jumping, kneeling, and playing. Joint-related disease, most notably arthritis, decreases the mobility of over forty million Americans. As the cartilage that allows the bones to move past each other breaks down, the joint can become too painful to move. If your joints are complaining to you through stiffness, swelling, aching pain, redness, or fever, consult your doctor for a formal diagnosis.

As you and your affected joints work together for more mobility, you'll find that moderate exercise can be of great benefit. Subject to your doctor's approval, stretching and endurance exercises can keep muscles around the joints strong and flexible, can help to decrease inflammation by increasing circulation, and can give you a more positive outlook. Celebrate your joints by moving them gently, slowly, and with love in your heart.

Assess Your Stress

What one has to do usually can be done.
—Eleanor Roosevelt (1884-1962)

A friend of mine shared with me how she and her husband survived moving to a new city and starting new jobs. She said, "We made a list of everything we had to do. Then we went back over the list and crossed off all the items we felt obligated to do, but weren't absolutely necessary. We cut that list by a third!"

I'm a list maker too. Sometimes it seems like there just are not enough hours in the day to accomplish all the things on my list. Feeling short on time, I'm soon agitated with unwanted adrenaline pouring into my system. But when I say, "There is enough of whatever I need," I see several of the items on my list don't really need to be done, or at least not done by me. Usually, I've taken responsibility for more than is my fair share, and in doing so, I've created a no-win situation for myself. Who takes the brunt of this poor decision-making? My body, of course.

Are you trying to do too much in too little time? If so, how is stress affecting your body today? Get out your body journal and find a clean sheet of paper. Draw an outline of your body and then color in the areas of your body that are carrying stress. Your middle back may be aching, your jaw may be clenched, the bottom of your feet may be tight. Mark all the areas you notice.

Now compare this month's drawing with last month's drawing. Are you carrying stress in similar places? Do you have any new locations? Are parts of your body more relaxed than last month? Keep your drawing so that you can see how stress affects you on a long-term basis.

Thank a Girlfriend

Friendship, like love, is the most important bread and butter for life.
—ANGNA ENTERS

My relationships with women can be so nourishing. They help heal the damage caused when I feel my body isn't acceptable in some way. For example, I was traveling on a speaking tour with a friend of mine, a beautiful woman with full, luscious lips. Mine are very thin and I have received the message that thin lips are unacceptable. I commented about this to my friend, almost under my breath, and she smiled at me and said, "There are lots of gorgeous women in the world with thin lips."

I said, "Name one."

She said, "Audrey Hepburn."

It was a short conversation. I don't even know if she remembers it now. But that moment of kindness helped me immensely. When I'm putting on my lipstick and feeling inferior because of the width of my lips, I smile now and comfort myself with my friend's words and Audrey Hepburn's image in my mind.

We've all had friends like this, who love us and help us expand our ideas of beauty and self-acceptance. Today, ponder how a girlfriend has helped you be more accepting of your body. And maybe give her a call and say, "Thanks!"

Leave the Wounds Behind

[T]he motor for our lives is within us, regardless of our past.
—CHRISTIANE NORTHRUP, M.D., *Women's Bodies,*
Women's Wisdom (1994)

I'm often asked by my clients to help them find out if pain they suffer is "emotional" or "physical." Steeped in traditional Western medicine, many of us view emotions as completely separate from the body. But research is disproving this notion, showing a link between what we feel emotionally and how we feel physically.

The relationship between body and emotions is complex, and we are far from understanding its intricacies. It would be a mistake, and self-abusive, to blame your feelings for your physical illness. At the same time, we are not helpless victims of our physical selves. I believe that by learning more about how your body communicates, you can cooperate and even expedite the healing process.

If you are suffering from an illness, discuss your concerns not only with your doctor but also with your body. I recommend using a technique called Active Imagination, usually applied to an inner dialogue between yourself and a dream figure. If you have a computer, type out your questions in lower case. Allow your body to respond to you in upper case. If you don't have a computer, writing the dialogue longhand works just as well.

Ask your body what the pain means. Let your body answer. You may find out some vital information that will help you leave the emotional wounds behind. Emotional healing may help you better cope with the illness and, perhaps, lead toward healing the problem altogether.

Be Compassionate with Yourself

Self-nurturing means, above all,
making a commitment to self-compassion . . .
—JENNIFER LOUDEN, *The Woman's Comfort Book* (1992)

In one of the women's groups I facilitate, a participant, Jenny, discussed her fear of expressing sadness in front of the others. "I'm afraid that it's wrong to cry here, afraid that you'll be upset with me." In previous weeks, Jenny had demonstrated deep compassion for another woman in the group who had cried while discussing a past experience. I was struck by how effortlessly Jenny honored the vulnerability of another woman while believing her own feelings were unacceptable. I've been guilty of this belief myself. It is easier for me to feel compassion for other women than for myself, easier to accept the bodies of other women than my own.

In his day, Jesus said we're to love our neighbors as ourselves. For today's woman, I believe he would have said, "Love yourself with the same compassion you love others." Would you expect a friend to go to work when she's sick with the flu? Give yourself permission to care for yourself the next time you get sick. Do you reject your loved ones when they need a hug? Open yourself up to the affection you need today. Are you concerned about what your children eat, wanting them to get nutritious meals? Treat yourself to fresh fruits and vegetables. Give your body the same respect you give the bodies of the people you love.

Prepare for Romance

We can perhaps learn to prepare for love. We can welcome its coming,
we can learn to treasure and cherish it when it comes, but we cannot
make it happen. We are elected into love.
—IRENE CLAREMONT DE CASTILLEJO

Valentine's Day is approaching, no doubt triggering thoughts and images of romantic love. If you are in a loving relationship, you're probably anticipating the fourteenth happily. If you're in-between relationships, the thought of spending a romantic holiday alone may leave you a bit depressed, sadly pondering the pluses and minuses of past romances. No matter what your romantic situation may be this year, your body needs and deserves your love and attention. So take a few moments out of your day and enjoy a romantic bath shared by you and your body.

Play a tape of the most romantic music you can find to set the mood. Light a couple of candles, and turn out the lights. In the flickering light, disrobe, letting your clothes drop seductively onto the floor, and slip your gorgeous naked body into a silk wrap. Pin one red rose in your hair.

Drawing the bath, pour two to three cups of powdered milk into the water. After the bath is full, sprinkle rose petals across the water. Sink into the bath, knowing that your skin will be cleansed and healed by the milk bath. Ahhh. . . . Let yourself be surrounded by the sensuous warmth. Imagine your romantic fantasy.

After you have soaked awhile, cleanse your skin with a rose-scented, gentle soap. Rinse and softly towel yourself dry. You and your body are refreshed and ready for romance, whatever form it may take.

Locate Love in Your Body

Love and Reason, like a Fever and Ague,
took their alternate Turns in my Breast. . . .
—MARY HEARNE, *The Female Deserters* (1719)

I saw her standing at my door, but at first I didn't recognize her. In spite of her fifty-plus years, Penny held herself like a teenager, eyes dancing, skin fresh and full of color. I barely invited her in before she announced what her body had already told me—"I'm in love!" she declared with glee.

Love is an emotion that pulses through our bodies with the power to transform us, renew us, remake us into more viable beings. We feel younger, more alive, more vibrant. Our hearts beat faster and our lungs breathe deeper. Loving and being loved is not merely an emotional experience; it draws our entire beings, especially our bodies, into the glorious celebration.

How does your body express love? Is there tingling in your tummy or down in your toes? Does your heart feel light? Your muscles relaxed and your spine straight and flexible? Locate love in your body today. After recording your findings in your body journal, go out and share some love with someone else. It's more fun that way.

Celebrate Your Orgasm

A healthy sex life. Best thing in the world for a woman's voice.
—LEONTYNE MARY PRICE, in *Untamed Tongues* (1993)

Orgasms not only feel good, they can make you healthier too! A recent oncology study found that women diagnosed with breast cancer had a higher survival rate if they enjoyed regular, frequent orgasms. The researchers compared women who had sexual partners with women who masturbated, and both groups had a better prognosis than women, with or without partners, who rarely experienced orgasm.

Who knows why? I don't, but I suspect that part of the physical benefit of orgasm is increased oxygen intake which has long been linked with better health and which has been found helpful in fighting cancer. So orgasms away, my sisters! You'll have more fun, and you just might live longer as well!

Happy Valentine's Day.

Set Your Boundaries

No one can build his security on the nobleness of another person.
—WILLA CATHER, *Alexander's Bridge* (1912)

Write in the numbers indicating how often, if ever, the statements are true. Modify those statements that don't apply to you. 1—Never, 2—Sometimes, 3—Always.

___I trust my body.

___I listen when my body says my boundaries are violated.

___My body helps me decide who is trustworthy and who is not.

___The people in whom I confide rarely, if ever, betray my trust.

___My boundaries are clearly defined in intimate relationships.

___I enjoy relationships without losing myself in others.

___I honor other people's boundaries.

___I take responsibility for my own sense of safety.

___I refuse to take responsibility for other people's feelings.

___I have a clear sense of who I am and where I am.

___I say "yes" when I want to say "yes."

___I say "no" when I want to say "no."

___I do not allow those in authority to control my choices.

___I am able to tell others when I feel hurt without blaming them.

___I receive massage from a therapist who honors my boundaries.

Scoring Evaluation

37-45   Great! You set and protect clear, flexible boundaries.

26-36   Watch out. Your boundaries aren't as clear as you need.

0-25   Body alert! Your boundaries are in need of major repair.

Define Yourself

*Women need to know that they can reject the
powerful's definition of their reality.*
—bell hooks, *Feminist Theory: From Margin to Center* (1984)

Who defines who you are? When I ask women why they dislike their bodies, their answers usually focus on the size or shape of their bodies. Some feel they're too fat, their breasts are too small, their thighs are too flabby or their toes are too long. Underneath this negative judgment lies a fear of being rejected by men.

Historically, women have been defined by their relationships with men as wives, daughters, sisters, mothers. Because of limited access to financial resources, our female ancestors were often dependent upon their bonds with men for survival. Being connected to a man who could provide protection and resources for a woman and her children was a priority. Consequently, women were judged and valued by how well they served men as cooks, homemakers, lovers, and companions.

Times have changed, but many women unconsciously live within the psychological confines of their foremothers. While we can now own property, gain access to financial success directly, and survive with or without men, many of us continue to define ourselves, especially our bodies, by standards set by men. Consequently, we live at the mercy of their perceptions.

Take back your personal power. Protect yourself against the destructive dangers of self-loathing by defining yourself. Assess yourself on your own terms. Are you genuinely dissatisfied with your body? You may find your shape quite pleasing, but have felt afraid to say so. Let your body be acceptable to you right now. You can do it. Your body will give you strength.

Cut the Caffeine

If I knew what I was so anxious about, I wouldn't be so anxious.
—MIGNON MCLAUGHLIN, *The Second Neurotic's Notebook* (1966)

I used to have intense panic attacks, waking up in the middle of the night with my heart pounding, convinced I was about to die. Eventually these episodes got so bad I went to the doctor. He told me he was willing to try medication, but first he wanted me to completely remove caffeine from my diet.

At the time, I rarely drank water. Except for breakfast, I drank caffeinated soda with every meal. Well, to be honest, I drank about three or four sodas at every meal and a couple more between meals and before I went to bed. I was thirsty, after all.

I did what the doctor said and stopped guzzling caffeine. Amazingly enough, the panic attacks stopped as well. I still miss soda from time to time, but I don't miss the panic attacks. It's definitely worth the trade for me.

How many caffeinated drinks do you have a day? If you're drinking one or less, you're in fine shape. But two or more is a few too many. Give your system a break and let it settle into a natural rhythm rather than depend on a chemical to keep you going.

Be Critical

Be critical. Women have the right to say:
This is surface, this falsifies reality, this degrades.
—TILLIE OLSEN, *Silences* (1978)

In her remarkable book, *Women's Bodies, Women's Wisdom*, Dr. Christiane Northrup quoted her father as saying, "Feelings are facts. Pay attention to them." Wise words from a wise man.

I know that there are times I can trust my feelings and other times I mustn't. If I'm out of sync with my body, emotions may reflect my interior pain rather than an external situation. I am damaged psychologically, physically, and spiritually when my body and I are at war. However, when I am deeply rooted in my body, I seem to know things about other people without being sure exactly how I know. With amazing accuracy, I sense their motives, their needs, their shadows. These are feelings and insights I can trust.

All too often, when women speak out we're dismissed as too emotional, having PMS, or bitchy. Sometimes these criticisms are warranted, if we are projecting our interior pain onto others. However, if you and your body are at peace, then your feelings are most likely a clear reflection of what is going on around you. Even if others are offended by your views, speak them clearly from an honest heart.

Come home to your body and trust your feelings. Both your body and your feelings are God's gifts to you for guidance, protection, and insight.

Speak without Saying a Word

The gesture is the thing truly expressive of the individual—
as we think so will we act.

—MARTHA GRAHAM, in JOHN HEILPERN, "The Amazing Martha,"
The Observer (1979)

One look at my cats and I know what they're feeling. A swish of Sassy's tail warns of a paw that will soon reach out and smack Stud on the side of the head as punishment for disturbing her afternoon nap. A dreamy look on Stud's face lets me know he wants affection. Without being able to talk, they communicate clearly.

As a culture, we place a much higher value on creatures who can talk than on those who don't. Certainly we view animals and infants to be "lower" than those who can put their feelings, thoughts, and ideas into words. Some have assumed that as infants cannot communicate verbally, they are unable to think at all. In fact, I was taught in graduate school that infants are unable to feel and certainly not able to remember until they develop verbal skills.

Researchers are now discovering that feelings and cognitive abilities develop with or without verbal capacities. Take pleasure in your nonverbal communication skills—the smile that says, "I love you," a handshake that welcomes a friend, an elbow poked in the ribs of a spouse that says, "Shh . . . don't say that!," or a sexy walk that purrs, "Come hither." Be aware of how many ways you tell others how you feel and what you want without saying a word.

Make a Date with Your Body

Any woman who has a career and a family automatically develops
something in the way of two personalities. . . . Her problem is to keep
one from draining the life from the other.
—Ivy Baker Priest, *Green Grows Ivy* (1958)

Most women today juggle a variety of demands and obligations, often in service to the needs of others. Even though I am single, I rarely have a free minute to spare between my personal life and professional duties. Either I'm meeting writing deadlines, seeing clients, and presenting workshops or I'm spending time with friends and family. It's very easy to overlook one of the most important relationships I have—the one with my body.

Whether you're married or single, with or without children, we all have relationships that we value and therefore require attention. Make sure that, along with scheduling time to take your daughter to ballet class, take soup by a sick friend's house, meet your partner for dinner, and attend the next committee meeting, you schedule time to relate to your body. Don't wait until your body has to get your attention by landing you in bed with illness or some other physical ailment.

Take out your date book and make a date with your body. Plan something fun and nurturing like a workout at the gym, soaking in a hot bubble bath, or a soothing massage. Even though others are competing for your time and attention, put your body on the top of your priority list. That's one relationship you can't live without.

Bathe in Hawaii

There must be quite a few things a hot bath won't cure,
but I don't know many of them.
—SYLVIA PLATH (1932-1963)

In the mood to go to Hawaii? You can travel there via your bath tub at a fraction of the cost with no jet lag! Imagine warm, humid breezes wrapping around your body as you look down the vine-covered cliff onto the beach below. The piercing blue sky is streaked with orange and pink as the sun begins to snooze. Clipping a gardenia from a bush by the door, go inside your thatched hut, and turn on the cassette tape, enjoying Hawaiian music as it fills the room. Cut a pineapple and a couple of oranges into circles, sprinkle them with dried coconut, and arrange the fruit on a plastic platter.

As your bath fills, pour in a generous portion of fruit bubble bath. Toss half of the pineapple and orange rings into the tub. The water is ready. Disrobe and sink slowly into the warm, sweet water. Closing your eyes, take in the sensations of Hawaii. Take three deep, luxurious breaths. "I love Hawaii!" you remind yourself. "I must come here more often." Slowly munch on the remaining fresh fruit. The sweetness delights your tongue. Ahhh. . . . What a wonderful place, and how fortunate you are to have traveled there today. It's time to return to the mainland, but you can take the magic of Hawaii with you. Once dressed, you pin the gardenia in your hair as a reminder of your trip. Aloha!

Tell

Silence is the door of consent.
—BERBER PROVERB

Don't tell! This command is common to all women who have been abused in any fashion and at any age. When I was robbed at gunpoint I was commanded to give over my purse, which I did. The assailant's words were predictable. He said, "Don't yell." Women's descriptions of being molested as young girls differ in the type of abuse, but what is common to all is the command, "Don't say anything." And most of us obey and live in silence.

Fortunately for us, God created our bodies so that they could not comply with someone's cruel demand for silence. Our bodies speak clearly and loudly about how we've been harmed. Research reveals that there is intelligence inside each cell, registering the terror, the sadness, the shock, and the pain. As we listen to our bodies, we hear our own stories. And as we allow ourselves to tell our stories to others who believe, healing is possible.

Give yourself permission to tell someone about a difficult experience. You may attend a support group, call your body buddy, or talk with your mate. Follow your body's lead, the part of you who refuses to comply with "Don't talk," and tell the truth.

Make Peace with Your Parents

My father was a proctologist, my mother an abstract artist.
That's how I see the world.
—SANDRA BERNHARD, Comedian

Our parents shape not only our outlooks on life, but the ways we view and value our bodies as well. Take out your body journal and describe how your parents viewed their bodies when you were growing up. Did they treat their bodies with respect by eating well, exercising regularly, and getting proper rest? Were they comfortable with expressing love physically? Were they happy with their bodies?

If you had limited contact with one or both of your parents, these questions may be difficult to answer. Whether your parents were present or absent, they influenced how you view your body today. Describe how you value your body. Do you routinely meet your body's basic needs such as ample rest, regular exercise, and proper nutrition? Do you protect yourself from the winter weather by wearing appropriate coats and shoes? Are you comfortable in your clothing? Do you feel good about your appearance?

Do you see any similarities between the way you relate to yourself and the way your parents treated their own bodies? Most likely you will. Underline those characteristics that strengthen your relationship with your body. And identify the ones you intend to change.

Eat More, Eat Less

The human organism needs an ample supply of good building
material to repair the effects of daily wear and tear.
—INDRA DEVI, *Renewing Your Life through Yoga* (1963)

I read recently that diet contributes to "about 60 percent of the cancers in women and about 30 to 40 percent of the cancers in men." To help strengthen our bodies against cancer, we need to eat more and eat less.

Eat more . . . apples.

Eat less . . . sour cream.

Eat more . . . broccoli.

Eat less . . . bacon.

Eat more . . . tomatoes.

Eat less . . . beef.

Today, follow the "more and less" idea for a healthier body. No need to feel deprived, simply eat more of the good foods!

Practice Waiting

Like an ability or a muscle, hearing your inner wisdom
is strengthened by doing it.
—ROBBIE GASS

Up, down, up, down, up, down. Repetition is required to strengthen a muscle. Similarly, hearing your body's guidance requires practice and repetition. For several months, I listed my intuitive impressions about what my body was telling me about myself in the present and how best to make decisions about my future. I discovered a curious thing. In every situation, I accurately picked up on the fact that my body was sending me some sort of message. Unfortunately, I drew inaccurate conclusions about what these messages meant about seventy percent of the time.

For example, I went to dinner with a friend and, as we walked into the restaurant, my shoulders tightened and I lost my appetite. Without talking with him, I concluded my body was telling me that he was angry with me. I feared his rejection so I withdrew. During dessert, he asked me if he had offended me. I informed him that he was the one who was angry, and then we both started laughing, realizing that we were both responding to stories we'd made up in our heads. For the first time that evening, we genuinely communicated. He told me how anxious he had been when he first came in the restaurant, sensing that I was unhappy with him for some reason. My shoulders and stomach had, indeed, sensed his emotional tension, but it was fear not anger.

I'm getting better and better at accurately interpreting my body's messages. But, like with any skill, it takes practice . . . and a little humility.

Enjoy a Normal Day

Normal day, let me be aware of the treasure you are. Let me not pass
you by in quest of some rare and perfect tomorrow.
—MARY JEAN IRION, *Yes, World* (1970)

I remember a time when I was never content. If I was with people, I'd long to be alone with my own thoughts. When I was by myself, the loneliness would overcome me, stirring up desire to be with someone, anyone. No matter what I was doing, I wanted to do something else. No matter what time of year it was, I longed for a different season. Living either in the past or the future, I missed the joys of living the day God had given me.

The more I've made peace with my body, the less I long to be somewhere else, doing something else at some other time. Past glories or future fantasies pale in comparison with the rich sensual realities of right now, right here. Wishing for tomorrow robs us of the flesh-and-blood experience of today.

Live today, today. And when tomorrow comes, live *that* today, today. Let living in the present become a normal experience by focusing attention on your body's sensations. Notice how your feet feel inside your shoes, how the heat from the fireplace warms your face, or how a cup of hot tea soothes you inside and out. Notice the little things, the often overlooked sensations that root us in the present.

Teach Body-Love to the Children

By the power of our imagination we can sense the future generations breathing with the rhythm of our own breath or feel them hovering like a cloud of witnesses. Sometimes I fancy that if I were to turn my head suddenly, I would glimpse them over my shoulder. They and their claim to life have become that real to me.
—JOANNA MACY, *The Way Ahead*

I believe that God gives each generation the opportunity to confront the mistakes of their ancestors and set things right. One of the most damaging beliefs I've inherited from those who have come before me is the separation of body from spirit.

We have a choice, a very important choice, to make. Will we pass this lie on to the next generation so that they, too, will suffer as we have, or will we do the work required to bring the body and spirit back into harmony? How will your struggle to make peace with your body impact the children in your life?

Teach body-love to children by the simple act of complimenting their bodies. Point out how healthy their skin looks today, how bright their eyes sparkle, how much you enjoy the music of their laughter, or how much you love their hugs. Let your compliments be sincere, and focus specifically on their bodies. You will give them a gift more valuable than gold.

Celebrate Your Eyes

Maybe a way of seeing all of life more fully
is to start by marveling at our own eyesight.
—CARL KOCH AND JOYCE HEIL, *Created in God's Image* (1991)

Do you take your eyes for granted? I do. My eyesight is fairly good, and until I reached forty, I didn't need glasses. Consequently, I've not had to think about my eyes very often. I just use them, assuming they'll always be there to help me. Except, that is, until I get a migraine headache, which starts with a "visual disturbance," a technical name for losing part of my eyesight. Little spots appear, somewhat like after having several flash pictures made. When I see those spots, I know I have about thirty minutes before the pain begins.

Migraines are no fun, regardless of where I might be. But headaches are easier managed when at home, near medication, stretched out on my own bed, complaining to a sympathetic friend on my own telephone. The problem is that not being able to see properly can make it quite difficult to drive home, find my medication, or even locate the bed. If I'm in town somewhere, I might have to call upon a friend to come rescue me and get me to a place where I can be miserable for several hours. At those time I really value my eyesight.

Take out your body journal and describe two or three experiences you have had that remind you to appreciate the marvel of eyesight. Then write your eyes a thank you letter in your journal so that your eyes can read it anytime.

Be in Your Body

Mr. Dufy lived a short distance from his body.
—JAMES JOYCE (1882-1941)

Years ago I was in a car accident in which no one was hurt, but my car landed in a young family's front yard. Looking back on that experience, I watch myself behind the wheel as a truck in front of me swerves unexpectedly. More like an observer than a participant, I see my car spin out of control and land on the lawn.

While feeling separated for a short time when traumatized can be helpful in surviving the experience, this approach to self-protection can actually place us in more danger if we stay out of touch with ourselves. If we are disconnected from parts of ourselves, we no longer have access to all of our emotional, intellectual, and physical resources. The more present we can be, the more able we are to notice warning signs and adequately protect ourselves from harm. The safest path is one taken fully present in your body, with both feet firmly walking on the ground.

Ground yourself by taking off your shoes and walking barefoot. Shuffle your feet on the floor so that your soles feel alive. Let the ground hold your weight as you balance your weight equally over each leg. The next time you feel disconnected from your body you can use this simple exercise to reconnect to the earth. Once grounded, you are best equipped to protect yourself.

MARCH

POCKETS

I don't have a proper
pocket,
none large
enough to carry
your kindness
and respect.
Your generous gifts
slip awkwardly
from my hands
as I fumble for a place
to keep them.
I need to
sew me some
Captain-Kangaroo-
way-down-deep-pockets
big enough
to hold
your love.

Create Safe and Nurturing Relationships

Do not protect yourself by a fence, but rather by your friends.
—Czech Proverb

I ask all my clients to promise me that if they ever feel pain during a massage session, they will tell me. I tell them that while I cannot promise they'll never feel pain, I can promise that as soon as I am aware of it, I will change what I'm doing. And then I tell them, "This is the best deal you can expect from a relationship. No one can promise not to hurt you. But those in your life can promise to respond to you once you communicate your pain to them."

Some of my clients readily tell me when I'm pressing too deeply into a muscle or when I've moved into a tender place during the session. But most of the women I work with find it difficult to tell me when it hurts. We have been taught that it is better to endure pain than to inconvenience anyone else. In spite of my request to tell me the truth, some women secretly fear I'll be angry with them for making their needs known.

How we relate to our bodies and physical pain often parallels how we relate emotionally to those around us. Women who have difficulty telling me that their shoulders are sore or the arch of their foot hurts when I press also have difficulty telling their spouses of emotional pain or identifying unmet intimacy needs. If we fear emotional or physical punishment in response to our asking for gentler handling or nurturance, we'll probably suffer our emotional wounds in silence.

Do you feel safe in your relationships? If you are not sure, observe your body the next time you are with a friend, spouse, or family member. Your body will tell you the truth about the relationship, so trust your gut.

While your conscious mind is trying to figure out what's what, your stomach and brain are communicating to each other through a network of nerve cells. Michael Gershen, M.D., chairperson of the department of Anatomy and Cell Biology at Columbia College of Physicians and Surgeons, claims that in anxiety-producing situations, "the brain can tell the entire system to speed or slow the digestive system." So sophisticated is this nerve system (it's more extensive than the spinal cord), Dr. Gershen says the stomach "too has a brain." The safer you feel in the relationship, the more relaxed and comfortable your stomach will be.

Your body will also tell you when someone who is usually trustworthy has unintentionally violated your boundaries or hurt you in some way. Use your voice to speak up and say, "Ow, that hurt." Safe people respond by altering their behavior, offering you nurturance rather than criticism.

Follow your body. Trust your gut. You will be led to safe and nurturing people. Your body knows.

Jog Safely

*The problem with jogging is that by the time you realize
you're not in shape for it, it's too far to walk back.*
—RODNEY DANGERFIELD, Comedian

A re you diligently jogging to keep fit? Great, but be careful that
you also keep yourself safe in the process. To help motorists
see you, especially after dark, wear reflective tape on your clothing
and shoes (front and back). Also, don't jog in the road. Stay on the
sidewalk or shoulder of the street, and run facing the traffic so you
can see who is approaching you.

Another hazard for joggers is the potential of being mugged or
raped. Safety experts claim that jogging with a dog greatly reduces
the risk of being attacked, especially if the dog is medium to large
in size. If you don't own a dog, you might borrow one from a friend.
Or you might even rent a dog. Your community may have a program
similar to one in Eugene, Oregon, called Project Safe Run. Founded
by Shelly Reecher, Project Safe Run provides dogs at a nominal fee
for walking and jogging purposes. Since its founding in 1981, their
dogs have accompanied over nine thousand runs without a single
incident!

Look and See

To see clearly is poetry, prophecy, and religion, all in one.
—JOHN RUSKIN, *Modern Painters*

Look at your body in the mirror and what do you see? Flaws? Cellulite? Stretch marks?

Now look at your body through the eyes of love. The picture will change. You'll see hands that give love to those you touch. An abdomen that tenderly holds your organs in place. Eyes that are wise from life's triumphs and pain. Knees that bend so you can look a small child in the eyes. Feet that take you on wonderful adventures.

Close your eyes to the superficial vision of our critical society. Open the eyes of love, and you'll see your body clearly, perhaps for the first time.

Laugh

A joyful heart is good medicine,
But a broken spirit dries up the bones.
—PROVERBS 17:22, *New American Standard Bible*

When I was a social worker dealing with child sexual abuse, I purchased a yearly pass to the local comedy club. Every Tuesday evening, nearly halfway through my week, I sat sipping my ginger ale and laughing until my sides split. I believe that one of the reasons my body held up under the stress of that job was my weekly dose of joy. It released stress from my body both through the spasm of laughing and through the chemical strengthening of my immune system.

Laughter has been proven to increase our bodies' ability to prevent disease and do battle with illness present in our systems. In addition, laughter is an enjoyable way to lose weight. According to William F. Fry, M.D., a psychiatrist at Stanford Univeristy School of Medicine, laughing one hundred times burns the same amount of calories as ten minutes on a rowing machine. So, go out of your way to laugh today. Rent a funny video, go to a comedy club, or ask a particularly witty friend out for dinner. Laugh. It will do your body good.

Explore Your Adolescence

Girlhood . . . is the intellectual phase of a woman's life, that time when, unencumbered by societal expectations or hormonal rages, one may pursue any curiosity from the mysteries of a yo-yo to the meaning of infinity. These two particular pursuits were where I left off in the fifth grade when I discovered a hair growing in the wrong place and all hell broke loose.

—ALICE KAHN

Our bodies take us into adolescence whether we are ready emotionally or not. I remember starting the fifth grade as a cute little girl and emerging as a gangly adolescent. At the age of ten, I sprouted up to my current five-foot, six-inch frame, staring down at the tops of my classmates' heads (especially the boys). I swear I could stare at my feet during class and watch them grow to a monstrous size nine and a half. My face exploded with red bumps that made me want to hide for the next ten years. I and my body awkwardly stumbled toward womanhood, all hands and feet with no curves. I felt too tall, too skinny, too zitty.

Often our opinions of ourselves as women are rooted in how we felt about ourselves during our adolescent years. Women who felt good about themselves as teenagers are more likely to have high self-esteem as adults. And the reverse is also true.

Take out your body journal and draw a picture of yourself when you were in junior high school, including those parts you were proud of and those that made you cringe. Describe how you felt about yourself when you first discovered the changes in your body. How do these feelings affect you today?

Celebrate Your Legs

How beautiful are your feet in sandals,
O prince's daughter!
The curves of your hips are like jewels,
The work of the hands of an artist.
—SONG OF SONGS 7:1, *New American Stanadard Bible*

In my practice, I see quite a few legs up close, and I work with many women who suffer from varicose veins. Most express embarrassment over how their legs look, often wishing to hide their legs from view. Short of having these veins surgically removed, we can minimize both the visual and physical discomfort of varicose veins by giving our legs more support and attention.

Sit more often than stand, but when you are standing wear support nylons. When sitting, resist the urge to cross your legs and prop up your feet whenever you can. Altering your diet can help, too. Eat more high-fiber foods, since constipation increases the likelihood of developing varicose veins, and decrease your salt intake to prevent retention of water and swelling. Movement increases circulation, so even if you're stuck in the office, sitting on a plane, or restricted in some other situation, gently rotate your ankles and stretch your toes.

Your legs deserve good circulation, proper exercise, and your admiration.

Assess Your Stress

Things could be worse. Suppose your errors were counted and published every day, like those of a baseball player.
—ANONYMOUS

While at times it may seem like the whole world is watching our every mistake or criticizing each of our blunders, few of us (thank goodness) have our pictures on the covers of magazines near the grocery store checkout stand. I used to be concerned about what other people were thinking, until I realized that most of them were thinking about themselves, not me! So, why get stressed out?

How is your stress level? Are you worrying about what other people are saying about you? It's time to assess your stress and see if you need to let go of outside pressure.

Get out your body journal. Using a blank page, draw an outline of your body and color in the stress points. Your hands may cramp, your scalp may constrict, or your ankles may ache. Mark all the areas throughout your body, and note if these sensations are being caused by criticism from others.

Compare this drawing with those you've drawn before. Trends and patterns may be more apparent after you've done this exercise for several months. But be open to surprises. Bodies are continually trying to communicate to us, and a new part may tense up just to get our attention. If you feel comfortable, share your drawings with your body buddy or someone else you trust. What does your body buddy notice?

Accept the Limits of Embodied Intimacy

To mature is in part to realize that while complete intimacy and omniscience and power cannot be had, self-transcendence, growth and closeness to others are nevertheless within one's reach.
—SISSELA BOK, *Secrets* (1983)

As pre-born babies, we floated in a private sea completely immersed in our mothers' bodies. Birth ended those blissful days, although some of us refuse to accept that we'll never recapture our womb experience. We may try to recreate a sense of total connectedness with our romantic partners. Since sex brings another body close to us and may bring a loved one inside us, we may hope to reexperience our pre-birth state. But romance and sex cannot carry the weight of this unrealistic expectation. If we expect to feel surrounded and held, like we once were in our mothers' wombs, we will be sadly disappointed.

Coming to grips with this fact can be painful, even agonizing. But the death of this dream makes way for the birth of a new possibility—that of knowing another person and of being known. Intimacy, especially sexual intimacy, is a body-rich experience, where touching and sensing take over where talking leaves off. As you draw as close as you can to the person you love, your body will communicate powerfully, perhaps more powerfully than all the words you long to say.

Stop Smoking

Do you have trouble blowing out the candles on your birthday cake?
Do you get winded dashing up a short flight of stairs?
—DON R. POWELL, *365 Health Hints* (1990)

Even though the dangers of smoking are common knowledge, more than fifty million Americans still smoke. Cigarette smoking is said to be responsible for over 390,000 premature deaths each year through heart disease, emphysema, strokes, and, of course, cancer. If you smoke, it's time to make changes. Today.

If you can, quit cold turkey and never look back. If that won't work for you, try this gradual plan. Get out your calendar and mark the date one week from today—your official quitting day. For the next week, keep track of every cigarette you smoke in your body journal. Save the butts in a jar so you get an honest look at all the cigarettes you're smoking.

On your quitting day, get rid of *all* your cigarettes and smoking aids. Substitute something healthy during the times you used to smoke like walking, talking to friends, chewing gum, drinking water—anything that keeps you from smoking. If possible, stay away from sugar and caffeine. Hang on. In about three months the urge to smoke will subside. You may always be attracted to smoking, but you'll notice new benefits as your system detoxifies. Food will taste better, your breath will be sweeter, and you'll breathe easier. Toss out the cigarette butts and put the money you would have spent on cigarettes in the jar. Once you fill the jar, grab your body buddy and the cash and celebrate.

Enjoy Solitude

If one says: I cannot come because that is my hour to be alone, one is considered rude, egotistical, or strange. What a commentary on our civilization, when being alone is considered suspect.
—ANNE MORROW LINDBERGH

What frightens us about solitude? I used to run from solitude, fearful of what I would hear in the silence. I kept music blasting on the radio, made sure I always had someone to eat with, and committed myself to projects that kept me busy every minute of the day. Finally, in 1985, my body insisted I be still by becoming ill and landing me in bed. My life came to a screeching halt.

With the help of my therapist, prayer group, body worker, and a few committed friends, I learned how to spend time with myself, listen to myself, love myself. Not that the process has been easy. Not at all. I was afraid to find out what was inside of me and, at times, craved some way to escape myself. But now, I can say that I genuinely relish solitude. I have confronted many demons, and now the silence doesn't frighten me. I know that when more issues arise for me to face, I will be successful, have the strength to resolve them.

Don't wait until your body makes a similar demand on you. Have courage and take time today for solitude. In the quiet, ask your body what message you need to hear today. Just be still and listen. Then record the message in your body journal.

Bathe in Spring

Spring comes: the flowers learn their colored shapes.
—MARIA KONOPNICKA, "A Vision" (19th Century) in JOANNA BANKIER
AND DEIRDRE LASHGARI, EDS., *Women Poets of the World* (1983)

Birds are singing. Light green leaves adorn branches that recently stood bare against the gray, winter sky. Buds pop out, promising colorful flowers soon. Rebirth is in the air.

All of creation goes through death and resurrection experiences. We let go of a hurtful relationship, making room for new love. We end a job that stifles our creativity and risk a new venture. Rejecting old images of our bodies, we insist on loving ourselves more.

Join the spring festivities. Acknowledge your personal rebirth by enjoying a refreshing bath. To prepare, find several sprigs of honeysuckle with its joyous aroma. Placing one sprig in your hair, save the other sprigs for your bath.

Play uplifting music that creates a sense of anticipation. After turning on the water in the tub, mix in a cup of oatmeal. This natural cleanser will gently remove the dead cells of the past and reveal your fresh new skin. Sprinkle the remaining sprigs of honeysuckle across the water.

As you sink into the tub and relax, picture the ending of some aspect of your life. Feel the sadness and grief, the tiredness and relief. Then imagine new birth, as your life now has room for more life and adventure. Let yourself be absorbed in the gladness as your lungs draw in the sweetness of the honeysuckle.

Wash yourself with gentle soap, removing all traces of the past. Rinse and gently pat yourself dry. Wear the honeysuckle in your hair the remainder of the day to remind you that you've passed through a valley of darkness and again into the light.

Locate Hope in Your Body

Hope is a very unruly emotion.
—GLORIA STEINEM, *Outrageous Acts and Everyday Rebellions* (1983)

A good friend of mine once said, "Hope is being open to the possibility of joy." I like that definition. Hope keeps us from plummeting into despair, the fine thread that pulls us out of bed each morning willing to invest in another day. Our bodies can experience hope as a force that propels us into an unknown future, overriding our imagined worst outcomes.

From time to time my hope for healing wavers. I feel unlovable, no matter what anyone around me may say or do. My hopelessness seems so real it overtakes my body, like a heavy weight across my chest and a limpness in my legs.

But when I feel lovable, hopeful for new experiences of intimacy, my body springs to life. Breathing is easy. My legs vibrate with enthusiasm. I am open, emotionally and physically, to the good that may come my way.

How does your body express hope in being loved? As a flickering smile, an urge you feel in your stomach, a bolt of energy in your fingertips? Take a good look at yourself today and locate hope in your body. Record your hopeful observations in your body journal. Be open to joy. Be open to love. Be hopeful.

Massage Your Face

Nature gives you the face you have when you are twenty. Life shapes the face you have at thirty. But it is up to you to earn the face you have at fifty.
—COCO CHANEL, in MARCEL HAEDRICH, *Coco Chanel: Her Life, Her Secrets* (1972)

Do your part in creating a beautiful face by relieving tension that causes lines to appear, and increasing circulation for better color and skin vitality.

Start at your forehead, rubbing your entire face with your fingertips. Along the way you may find sore spots. Give these a bit more attention.

Slowly open your mouth as far as it can go, feeling a stretch in your jaw muscles. Repeat until you can open your mouth fully and easily without pain. You may find yourself yawning or sighing as your body requires more oxygen to cleanse your facial tissues.

Lastly, reward yourself by caressing your face with your fingers, starting at the jaw line and working up. Be careful not to stretch your facial skin. Massage gently, communicating love and acceptance to your face.

Be Aware, Be Active

*Two things have happened to make people more fearful. First, there is
no longer the widespread belief that police and courts can protect
you. . . . The second thing is that the character of crime has changed.
Crime is teen-age, it's impulsive, it's irrational. Doing injury is the
purpose. . . . It's like getting hit by lightening.*
—GERALD M. CAPLAN, *Los Angeles Times*

Awareness and action are two themes I stress in my workshops.
Protecting our bodies from violence requires that we increase
our awareness about danger and then take new action.

To be safer, we must be more aware. Until I was personally
assaulted, I resisted being aware. While watching TV news reports
of violence, I comforted myself by saying, "That didn't happen
near here," or "I wouldn't have been in a situation like that." Facing
the fact that I am vulnerable to violence is an upsetting prospect,
one I'd rather ignore.

Sadly, it's quite possible that you or a woman you know may be
physically harmed in some way in the coming year. We will be
safer, not by pretending we're not in danger, but by becoming
realistically aware of what the dangers are. Overcome the first
obstacle to awareness by confronting the fear that may lull us into
pretending it could only happen to someone else.

Second, take action by contacting your local police department
and getting involved in a Neighborhood Watch or other crime
prevention program in your area. Resist the urge to turn your head
the other way. The head you protect may be your own.

Picture Yourself

I cannot express or represent myself without
the participation of my body.
—KARL BARTH, Theologian

If someone pointed to a photo of a little girl and asked, "Who is this?" our response may be, "That's Annie when she was five, the year we took a trip to the lake." We equate a picture of someone's physical form to be synonymous with who that person is. We would not say, "Oh, that's Annie's body when she was five years old."

You *are* your body. Take a look at a recent picture of yourself. What do you see? A "body" or a person? Look beyond the surface appearance (and if you look "good" or not) and see what your body tells you about yourself. How are you standing, erect or slouched? Are you touching anyone else? Is anyone touching you? Do you seem comfortable or tense? Are you smiling with your whole face or just with your mouth? Is your hair shining and healthy or dull and depressed? Record your observations in your body journal.

Show the picture to your body buddy to discover what she sees in the picture. You will find that your body conveys more than you might imagine.

Be a Juicer

If you want to be healthier, recover from illness, have more energy, and slow the aging process, eat more fresh, raw vegetables and fruit.
—CHERIE CALBOM AND MAUREEN KEANE, *Juicing for Life* (1992)

I was very excited about my new juicer, so I mixed up a concoction of kale, spinach, broccoli, and carrots. Certain this brew would lead me to immediate health, I downed the glass with enthusiasm. Ugh. . . . It tasted horrible and burned all the way down to my stomach. I felt it hit my stomach bottom, and with the same enthusiasm that the juice had gone down, it came right back up!

Even though my introduction to juicing was unpleasantly memorable, I still juice. Only I've learned to pay more attention to my body and less attention to recipes that suit other people's insides. Here's one of my favorite recipes that you may enjoy.

Juice together:

♦ Two large carrots.

♦ Three large peeled and seeded oranges.

♦ A handful of seedless grapes.

♦ Pour it into a tall glass and garnish with a sprig of mint.

This mixture is a good source of vitamin C and beta carotenes, both antioxidants that protect your cells from wear and tear. Bioflavonoids from the grapes help vitamin C's effectiveness. And it even tastes good! But remember to sip a little at first to make sure your tummy likes this as well as mine does.

Be a Witness

If I have one duty in these times, it is to bear witness.
—ETTY HILLESUM, Dutch Jew who died in Auschwitz,
November 30, 1943

Our bodies bear witness to what has happened to us in the past and what is occurring in the present. Imagine how valuable we must be to God for our bodies to be designed as historical records. Past injustices, wounds, and abuses are important to God, so important that our bodies remember through every bodily system: physical scars, muscular tension, skeletal construction, neurological patterning, respiratory functioning, hormonal balances, and conscious and unconscious memory.

Especially in difficult times, the body bravely records our sadness, fear, anger, and turmoil. Your joints may remember the weight placed on you as a child and your breathing pattern may speak of anxiety. A clenched jaw may reveal unexpressed anger, while a tilted pelvis perhaps speaks of sexual abuse. Hearing the message of the body can be painful, but it is critically important. Your story is an important one, one valued by God.

Our bodies speak truth in such a profound and powerful way that, I believe, learning to hear the message from our bodies parallels hearing God's voice. Listen and you'll hear that you are valuable beyond measure.

Be Radical

Women may be the one group that grows more radical with age.
—GLORIA STEINEM, *Outrageous Acts and Everyday Rebellions* (1983)

When I turn fifty I'm going to dye my hair blond. There, I've put it in print. Now I'll *have* to do it! The older I get, the less I worry about what people think and the more I'm willing to do outrageous things, wear clothes I like even if they are out of fashion, and speak my mind. I've got a few more years before I'll be feisty enough to go blond, but I am headed in the right direction.

Pick something outrageous to do today. You might need to find a daring girlfriend to join you on an escapade. Protest an injustice. Dress up in wild outfits and go dancing. Rent roller blades and skate the avenue. It doesn't have to be public, but it's more fun if it is. Go for it.

Accept the Limits of Cosmetic Surgery

Change is an easy panacea. It takes character to stay in
one place and be happy there.
—ELIZABETH CLARKE DURAN

Many women are having plastic surgery on those parts of their bodies with which they have not made peace. Rather than asking the question, "Is plastic surgery okay?" for yourself or other women, I believe the more important question to ask is, "How will you make peace with your body after plastic surgery?"

No matter how perfect the procedure, every woman who has cosmetic surgery still has a less-than-perfect body. Tummies may be tucked, but what about the legs? Or the breasts may be larger (or smaller), but what about the wrinkles around your eyes? The face may be tighter, but what about the veins in your legs? Surgery may relieve the stress caused by one part of the body, but no medical procedure can rescue us from having to make peace with our bodies as a whole.

Clients who ask me about plastic surgery receive my support in finding their own conclusions. I am neither for nor against it. What I *am* for is accepting ourselves as we are, no matter how we are. That process will be required of us regardless of having a tuck, a lift, or a strip. The challenge before us remains the same.

Celebrate Spring, Welcome Your Body

The air one breathed was saturated with earthy smells,
and the grass under foot had a reflection of blue sky in it.
—WILLA CATHER, *Death Comes for the Archbishop* (1927)

How does the coming of spring awaken us from winter's hibernation and bring us back to our senses? We tremble as spring's warm breezes tease and caress our skin and fill our lungs with the hope of new birth. The fresh fragrance of thawed soil and budding flowers tantalizes our nostrils. Freeing our feet from heavy boots and thick stockings, our toes delight once again in the softness of grass. It is impossible to experience spring apart from our senses. To welcome spring, we must first welcome our bodies.

Run out to meet spring today. To celebrate the season of rebirth, you'll need your eyes to see the colors of the sunset, your nose to enjoy the fragrance of the roses, your mouth to taste spring raindrops on your tongue, your skin to feel the warming sun, and your ears to hear the song of the birds. Welcome your body. Celebrate spring.

Play

Playing alone or with others—a round of golf, an aerobics class, a soccer game, a tennis match—isn't just frivolous nonsense. Play creates balance. It's the safety net under the tightrope of modern life; it keeps us sane and functioning.
—DAPHNE ROSE KINGMA, *True Love* (1991)

Recently my friend, Lynn, called me up and asked me when I had taken a day off. Angrily I said, "Stop pressuring me! I can't deal with taking care of myself right now!"

Ever get so stressed out that taking care of yourself feels like just another stressor?

The times we need to nurture ourselves the most are often the very times we feel so overwhelmed that we can't find the time, energy, or wherewithal to give ourselves what we need. When we're stressed out, we're in either the agitated or flooded states and are no longer connected to our full cognitive, creative, or emotional capabilities.

Take a few deep breaths, connect to your body, and settle into the alert processing state. Now, brainstorm a pageful of ways you can nurture, soothe, and encourage yourself (including getting others to help you with these goals). Keep this in a drawer nearby, and the next time you are so stressed out you can't think straight, read your list and do at least one of the activities you've described. Plan ahead. We're all going to get stressed out from time to time. Why act like it's a big surprise?

Declare a Truce

It is more blessed to give than to receive, so give to yourself
as much as you can as often as you can.
—LaVerne Porter Wheatley Perry

How would you rate your relationship with your body? Shared annoyance? Delighted acceptance? Engaged in full-out war?

My relationship with my body has changed over the years. Prior to my burnout in 1985, I treated my body as a servant who had no legitimate needs. "If my body was stronger," I fumed to myself, "I wouldn't need so much rest and I could accomplish so much more." When I fell ill, which I did regularly, a sense of hopelessness overwhelmed me, "Why am I stuck in bed again with another flu or infection?" If I had listened for an answer to these questions, I might have learned something. But I wasn't really asking for information. I was busy blaming my body.

The relationship I enjoy with my body now is much different. While I'm still prone to overdo, I am less blaming and more open to conversation with my body. When I'm pushing too hard, my body has ways of getting my attention that are less dramatic or disruptive than landing me flat on my back in bed. Most of the time I listen. Not always. But more often than I did in the past.

If you are in a war with your body, wave the white flag today and declare a truce. Notice what your body needs. A quiet walk? A glass of fresh water? A sensuous bath? A soothing massage? Sign a peace treaty by giving your body whatever it needs today.

Protect Your Body from AIDS

*Our first step in defining our sexuality from the inside out is to
consider ourselves as sex subjects rather than sex objects.*
—CHRISTIANE NORTHRUP, M.D., *Women's Bodies,
Women's Wisdom* (1994)

No one wants to believe they could contract AIDS, but this disease is part of our lives and will probably continue to affect us for years to come. Claiming ownership of our bodies and our sexuality, making decisions that are right for us, can be a matter of life and death. Since there is no known cure, prevention is the only way to survive this disease.

The HIV virus is transmitted through body fluids such as semen and blood from an infected individual. The most obvious way to protect yourself from contracting the virus is by abstaining from sex with anyone who is HIV-positive. Since you may not know if someone is infected, avoid high-risk partners, including homosexual and bisexual men, heterosexual men you know or suspect have had multiple partners, and IV drug users. Limit your sexual involvement to one, monogamous partner. Unless you are sure that both of you are virus-free and you and your partner are monogamous, use a latex condom and a spermicide containing Nonoxynol-9. Do not participate in anal intercourse or other sexual activities that might tear the vagina, rectum, or other tissue. If you suspect you've been exposed to the virus, contact your doctor or your local health department. Confidential testing is available. And reach out to those who love you, to obtain the emotional support you need.

Listen to Your Story

The power of storytelling lies in its embodied truth. . . . Their bodies
remember what it is like to be a no-body
and what it is like to be some-body.
—CHUNG HYUN KYUNG, *Struggle to Be the Sun Again*

Historically, women from most cultures have been deprived access to education and the opportunity to directly influence perceptions of the dominant society. Only men retained this form of overt power. However, as our grandmothers gathered together to quilt, to can vegetables and fruit, and to share meals, they communicated ideas by telling each other their stories. Now we live in an age in which we can speak out more directly about who we are and what we feel.

I believe it is critical, however, not to misuse this opportunity of freedom to abandon our womanly skill of storytelling. Through generations, women carried their stories in their bodies, sharing them with those who would listen. Now that we have access to education and can write, speak, teach, and communicate, let's take this historically rare gift to tell our stories, our truth.

We give each other a priceless gift when we listen to other women tell their stories. Join a supportive women's group and share yourself with them. You are embodied truth. I encourage you to continue to learn the language of your body so that you can translate this wisdom clearly to all who have the ears to hear.

Take Credit for Your Beauty

You can take no credit for beauty at sixteen.
But if you are beautiful at sixty, it will be your own soul's doing.
—MARIE CARMICHAEL STOPES (1880-1958)

Some of my clients lament that as they grow older they feel they are losing their youthful beauty. For many people, aging represents loss.

For me, however, the opposite is true. I was not an attractive teenager. My face was covered with pimples, my body lacked shape, and I was depressed (though we didn't have a name for it back then). Through therapy, inner work, and body work I've come to terms with many of my emotional problems. To my delight, I'm enjoying the unexpected side benefit of feeling more physically attractive.

I'll admit that my skin isn't quite as youthful and that gray hairs are sprouting up all over. But in spite of these signs of age, I feel better about my appearance than I ever did at sixteen. I credit this feeling to my soul work. And I feel fine about acknowledging my accomplishments and enjoying the changes.

Can you see the positive impact of your inner work on your outer beauty? List in your body journal the ways you feel better about your appearance now than you did when you were younger. You'll most likely be surprised at how much you've improved through the years.

Survey the Intimacy in Your Life

[L]ove was the key to every good.
—DORIS LESSING, *A Proper Marriage* (1952)

Write in the numbers indicating how often, if ever, the statements are true. Modify those statements that don't apply to you. 1—Never, 2—Sometimes, 3—Always.

___I feel touchable.

___I attract people into my life who respect my boundaries.

___I enjoy close relationships with women.

___I enjoy close relationships with men.

___I trust friends to "be there" for me in times of stress or crisis.

___I am comfortable with the ways I hug others.

___I ask for what I need effectively and respectfully.

___I say "no" to touch that feels uncomfortable.

___I pay attention to my body's messages when I am close to others.

___I let some people closer than others depending on how I feel.

___I'm aware of my body sensations when neglected or violated.

___I express my feelings when I feel hurt, neglected, or violated.

___Once others make amends for their wrongs I release all negative emotion.

___I make amends whenever I violate the boundaries of others.

___I receive regular massage that nurtures and empowers me.

Scoring Evaluation

37-45   Great! You're developing safe, nurturing relationships.

26-36   Watch out. You're not adequately protecting yourself.

0-25   Body alert! You are at risk of being hurt or abandoned. Pay attention to setting and protecting clear boundaries.

Celebrate Your Bones

Healthy self-care begins with checking to see if you are meeting your basic needs and then working to fulfill them.
—JENNIFER LOUDEN, *The Woman's Comfort Book* (1992)

Think of all your bones do for you—hold you up straight so you can drive, surround your brain so it doesn't fall on the floor, give your favorite shoes something to hold onto, and keep you from rolling around like a jellyfish. Important functions!

Since our bones make our lives possible, it's important to pay attention to their needs. As we age, our bones lose density. This process is accelerated after the age of forty and for women who have reached menopause.

Celebrate your bones today by getting at least 1,000 milligrams of calcium if you are premenopausal or 1,500 milligrams of calcium if you are postmenopausal. If you aren't already getting the calcium you need on a daily basis, let today be the first day of your new regime.

Calcium is fairly easy to come by. Foods rich in calcium include low-fat dairy products, salmon, sardines, beans, bean sprouts, broccoli (isn't there *anything* wrong with broccoli?), kale, and sunflower seeds. If you try a calcium supplement, stay away from those derived from bone meal or dolomite. And don't overdo it. Don't exceed the recommended dose.

So grab a nonfat yogurt or a handful of sunflower seeds and celebrate your bones!

Prepare for a Carjacker

*Most power is illusionary and perceptual. You have to create an
environment in which people perceive you as having some power.*
—CARRIE SAXON PERRY, in BRIAN LANKER, *I Dream a World* (1989)

Carjacking is a relatively new and sometimes deadly crime that
is increasing in many communities. The time to decide how
to deal with a possible carjacking is right now, when you're safe and
sound. Don't wait to think through how best to protect yourself at
the moment you're confronted by a threatening person. Imagine
yourself in a carjacking, and make a plan now that will maximize
your power for self-protection.

In *Not an Easy Target*, Paxton Quigley suggests cooperating with
an armed carjacker as long as his requests are limited to demanding
your keys and your purse. Quigley suggests getting out of the car as
soon as possible and letting him have the vehicle. If you are forced
to drive the car, make sure you do not end up in a deserted area
where no one can help if the carjacker intends to seriously harm
you, perhaps through rape or even murder. So if you are driving
the car, some experts suggest being on the alert for a chance to
crash into another empty car or pole at low speed and jump from
the car as soon as possible. Hopefully, the crash will scare him off
or at least attract enough attention that he'll be unlikely to kill you
when he's surrounded by witnesses.

Even though a carjacker may have a weapon, if you are armed
with a preconceived plan and the element of surprise, you'll be
better equipped to outsmart his attempt to control you.

Don't Wait to Relate

*"Wait a minute, I'm not finished yet," was the impatient response
from my five-year-old daughter when I once tried to get her to leave
her coloring book and come to dinner. She is now a grown woman
with two children of her own. I hope she still feels that way.*
—RAY ANDERSON, *Self Care* (1995)

At times I think, "Why in the world am I writing such a book?
There's so much I have to learn about the mysterious
connection between body and soul."

And then I remember that what I have to share is not perfection
but process. A few years back, I refused to listen to anything my
body had to say. Now at least there's a conversation going on. That's
progress.

Are you aiming for perfection or process? It's important for all of
us to converse with our bodies. I am going to ask you to do an
exercise which may seem strange, but can be helpful in hearing
your body's wisdom. Get out your body journal and write down a
question you have for your body. The question can be anything
you are trying to puzzle out right now in your life, such as, "Should
I stay in a particular relationship?" or "Is it time for me to change
jobs?" With your non-dominant hand, record your body's answer.
Continue the conversation and see what you learn about each other.
Continuing the conversation is all any of us can do.

Stretch Your Calves

*The uneventful and commonplace hour is
where the battle is lost or won.*
—Maltbie D. Babcock

Think of how many hours, over the course of a lifetime, we spend standing in front of the mirror brushing our teeth. Certainly keeping your teeth and gums healthy is an important part of body care, so hopefully you are looking at yourself, foaming at the mouth, at least twice a day.

To make the most of these moments, follow the example of a woman I know who has a wonderful smile and great legs. She does toe lifts to strengthen her calves while brushing her teeth. She gets an extra little workout for her legs while maintaining good oral hygiene. What an easy way to stay in touch with the top and bottom of your body simultaneously!

Ask Your Body for an Opinion

Who that has reason, and his smell,
Would not among roses and jasmine dwell,
Rather than all his spirits choke
With exhalations of dirt and smoke?
—ABRAHAM COWLEY

When I was a little girl, my mother tried to explain war to me. She said that it was a horrible thing where many people died, and even those who survived often never fully recovered emotionally from it. I thought, "She can't be right. If it's this horrible, why would any adult do such a thing?"

I was much wiser then than I am now. I knew that if something hurt, I probably shouldn't do it. But now, as an adult, I make decisions that disregard my obvious physical needs, such as living in Los Angeles amid the smog, increasing crime, and relentless stress. I'm still learning how to include my body in decisions. At least now I am taking my body's needs into consideration.

Are you making major decisions about where you may live or work? Along with income or status, consider your body's needs. What is the air quality? The crime rate? Opportunities for exercise and recreational activities? The pace of life? Make sure there are benefits for your body where you work and live.

APRIL

BREAD MAKING

Sensuous ball
of satin white elastic
you are more than a lump-of-clay
you are a responsive, living thing
you stretch, yet hold yourself together
as I pull against your structure
you yield, then spring back with counterforce
as I press my weight against your mass
it is as if you know
I work you hard
to give you breath
that you might rise
to nourish life
in others.

Turn Stresses into Challenges

The non-stimulated animal will not only learn to respond in a manner ill-suited with actual danger, it will also learn to respond far more readily to less physical threats and to more innocuous psychological stresses.
—DEANE JUHAN, *Job's Body* (1987)

Somewhere between feeling so bored life's not worth living and so overwhelmed that you go screaming hysterically into the night is a level of stress that produces a healthy life. Too little stress actually impairs our ability to discern danger and cope with even the smallest disruption. Too much stress burns out our systems and can easily cut years off our life spans.

I've found it helpful to differentiate between "stresses" and "challenges." Challenges are problems that I need and am able to resolve. We all need challenges—physical challenges that help our bodies, especially our nervous systems, to grow; psychological challenges to teach us how to cope effectively with others; creative challenges to motivate us to develop our talents; spiritual challenges to motivate us to wrestle with questions of meaning, morality, and purpose. Challenges take a reasonable amount of energy, and we are rewarded once we've successfully overcome the obstacle.

Stresses, on the other hand, are problems that need resolution, but for some reason I am unable to manage them successfully or in a time-efficient manner. Often stress contains factors which are out of my control. For example, I become stressed when I try to write a book chapter in too short a time, when I feel responsible for controlling a friend's behavior (which I can't control, darn it all), or when I'm caught in traffic and can't make all these people get out of my way!

When we are stressed, we move into agitated or flooded states, thereby triggering our sympathetic nervous systems. Your body responds to stress as it would to any life-threatening danger, through fear and a potent explosion of chemicals and physical reactions to give you extra power. The outpouring of hormones, especially adrenaline, is so powerful that your blood literally changes direction, abruptly darting toward your hands and feet so that you can fight or flee. To give you that burst of energy needed to do battle or escape, your digestive juices turn their corrosive capabilities away from the food in your stomach and onto your own tissue. Your heart beats faster, and your brain screens out everything but the danger. Every cell focuses on survival.

An agitated or flooded state is desirable if you need to get out of the way of a speeding car or if someone has broken into your house and you have to defend yourself. But remaining in this state will burn your body out in no time.

Pay attention to your body. Notice when your pulse is racing, your breath is short, and you have trouble taking in what is happening in the room. These clues let you know that you're in an agitated or flooded state and that your central nervous system is being stressed.

To the best of your ability, turn stresses into challenges. Say "no" to unrealistic demands. Protect yourself from dangerous relationships by setting firmer boundaries or removing yourself altogether. Become a more creative problem-solver and find new ways to tackle an old problem. And don't forget to celebrate your successes. Include your body in the celebration because without your body, you'd enjoy no successes at all.

Schedule a Massage

The impersonality of life in the Western world has become such that we have produced a race of untouchables.
—Ashley Montagu, *Touching: The Significance of Skin* (1986)

B ack in the days when I lived solely in my head, I rarely touched anyone, and I certainly didn't like it when anyone tried to touch me. Definitely not a "huggy" sort of person, I preferred relating to others via conversation, preferably at a distance, perhaps with a table or some other tangible object between us.

My reluctance to be physically close to others was, perhaps, one of the reasons massage and body work were so effective for me. The touch I receive in massage and body work is very structured, professional, and safe. No worries about "where this might lead." The boundaries are clear, the expectations shared. I can predict, within reasonable parameters, in what ways I'll be touched.

If you, for whatever reason, feel apprehensive about touching or being touched by others, massage and body work may offer you an opportunity for healing and nurturance not available in typical interactions with friends, family, or even with a mate. Contact a certified professional in your area and make an appointment to allow more touch into your life. Let touch guide you back home to your body.

Celebrate Your Heart

My sorrow is beyond healing.
My heart is faint within me!
—JEREMIAH 8:18, *New American Standard Bible*

Every twenty seconds an American dies of a heart attack. An additional 600,000 people die each year of coronary artery disease. We have known that men tend to die at an earlier age due to heart attacks than women, but until recently, we haven't realized the role stress has played in this dynamic. As more and more women enter the work force and cope with similar stressors to what men have faced, the rate of heart attacks is increasing among the female population. When we are distressed, grieved, frustrated, and stressed out, our hearts become sick.

Take your heart's health seriously. If you smoke, quit. Schedule a checkup to find out if your blood pressure, weight, and cholesterol levels are within a healthy range. Find one way to decrease the level of frustration in your life. Do it for your heart's sake.

Assess Your Stress

He who laughs, lasts.
—Mary Pettibone Poole, *A Glass Eye at a Keyhole* (1938)

Have you laughed much lately, or has the everyday grind gotten you down? It's time to assess your stress again this month to see if your body is having fun or suffering from too much tension.

Get out your body journal and draw an outline of your body. Using colored pens or pencils, color in the tense, painful, or tight areas in your body. You may have a sinus headache, throbbing in your abdomen, or lower back pain. Mark in all the areas where you feel discomfort or soreness.

Compare this drawing with the previous ones. Is there a pattern developing? Are some areas of your body chronically affected by stress? Are new areas of your body being affected? If you choose, share your drawing with your body buddy to see if she can shed even more light on what your body is telling you about the stress in your life.

If your body is tense, invite your body buddy to join you for an evening at a comedy club or to come to your place to watch a funny video. It's time to laugh off some stress.

Declare Your Body as Your Own

For ages we have accepted responsibility for other adults. . . . If we are to be responsible to anyone, let it be to ourselves first.
—STEPHANIE COVINGTON AND LIANA BECKETT,
Leaving the Enchanted Forest (1988)

I recently took a workshop from Carolyn Braddock, a therapist who works with women trauma survivors from a body-oriented perspective. From time to time, as she worked with different women, she would ask, "Who does your arm belong to?" or "Whose leg is that?" Without hesitation, these women would answer, "This is my father's arm," or "My leg belongs to the woman who molested me."

Many of us do not feel ownership of our own bodies. We have given that power away to those who overwhelmed us with their needs, demanding that we use our bodies to take care of them and neglect ourselves.

As we make peace with our bodies, we must reclaim ownership of our bodies, not in a possessive but in a protective way. Today, look at yourself in the mirror and declare that each part of your body is your own. Say aloud, "This is my arm. This is my hand. These are my breasts. These are my genitals." Make your body yours.

Reward Yourself for Exercising

Instant gratification takes too long.
—CARRIE FISHER

We all know we should exercise. So why don't we all get our allotment each and every week?

"I exercise but don't feel any payoff!" That's my favorite excuse for not exercising. I want to do a couple of leg lifts and see instant change in my thighs. Do you have a similar complaint?

The truth is there are few things more important to your health than exercising regularly. Exercise can help us live longer by decreasing chances for developing cancer (the more oxygen cells receive the healthier they become), experiencing heart attacks (by strengthening heart muscles), or suffering a stroke (by lowering blood pressure). In addition, exercise can increase self-esteem by giving us a more attractive shape and a sense of accomplishment.

For some people the exercise itself is reward enough. If you're like me and need an extra boost, then give yourself a treat. Perhaps promising yourself a relaxing afternoon of reading will be the motivator for a month of regular exercise. Or sharing afternoon tea with a friend at the end of a strenuous week's workout. If exercise is really a chore, daily rewards may be necessary, like enjoying a small scoop of fat-free, low-calorie yogurt or taking a fifteen-minute nap in the middle of the day. The rewards I give myself depend on what suits my fancy. Do whatever it takes to get you stretching, hopping, lifting, curling, crunching, and sweating!

Follow Your Own Advice

Please give me some good advice in your next letter.
I promise not to follow it.
—EDNA ST. VINCENT MILLAY, *Letters* (1952)

I tend to slump my shoulders. I went to one massage therapist who said my slumped shoulders indicated I was trying to protect a broken heart. The next body worker said that I was carrying the weight of the world on my shoulders. A third massage therapist informed me that my hunched shoulders were a sign of fear.

Perhaps all three of these well-intentioned therapists were right. I've had my heart broken, I feel excessively responsible for others, and I find life to be scary at times. But I suspect that what is better learned from these encounters is that the first body worker was recovering from a broken heart, the second felt overly responsible, and the third was grappling with fear.

Only you and God can tell for certain what your body is trying to tell you. I recommend listening to the insights and advice of others. But do whatever is best for you, in spite of their input. Today, depend on what your body feels rather than what other people think your body feels. Let your body be your guide.

Go to Feelgoodallover

Taking joy in life is a woman's best cosmetic.
—ROSALIND RUSSELL, Actor

Ready for a fantasy? Grab your body journal, a pen, and a timer. Relax in a comfortable chair, breathe deeply several times, and imagine yourself traveling to the land of Feelgoodallover. At the border, the guard asks to see your papers, so you bring out your license, passport, and credit cards. But he shakes his head no.

He says, "We only let people into Feelgoodallover who feel good all over. We must have proof." He sets the timer, saying, "Sit. You have four minutes to list all the people you love and who love you back. Go!"

Quickly, list the people you love who love you in return. Next, describe all the ways these people help you feel good about yourself (especially your body): sharing a workout with your best friend, the back massage you received from your partner, the compliment received from a co-worker. Stop when the timer rings.

The guard says, "Now write all the things that make you feel good about yourself." As the timer is set for another four minutes, list your finest attributes: your long neck, quirky sense of humor, the way your hair falls naturally into curls, your generosity, quickness at solving crossword puzzles, the softness of your skin, the sexy way you dance. The list grows and grows.

Bing!

"Time's up!" the guard declares and picks up your lists. "This is fine work. You are welcome to enter Feelgoodallover. In fact," he grins mischievously, "you are already here!"

Locate Loneliness in Your Body

I never said, "I want to be alone." I only said,
"I want to be let alone." There is all the difference.
—GRETA GARBO, in JOHN BAINBRIDGE, *Garbo* (1955)

One of my clients described an agonizing loneliness, saying, "Even though I'm married and the house is full of kids, I can't shake the sense of being alone with no one really seeing me and noticing I'm hurting." Loneliness can strike no matter who else is around. Whether you live alone or with others, feeling isolated and unnoticed can cut deep into our souls and our bodies.

Some bodies bend under the weight of carrying life's burdens without support. Feet may drag, intestines may fill with gas, hair may lose luster. How does your body express loneliness?

The next time you feel lonely, ask your body buddy to observe your body's movements. Record your new awareness in your body journal. Talk to your body buddy about your feelings of loneliness. Before you know it, your loneliness may disappear.

Nourish Yourself Inside and Out

All happiness depends on a leisurely breakfast.
—JOHN GUNTHER (1901-1970)

Enjoy this morning with a breakfast that nourishes on the outside as well as on the inside. First, nourish yourself on the outside by enjoying a peaches-and-cream mask. Simply mash a soft, ripe peach in a bowl and add a tablespoon of cream. Mix thoroughly. Apply to your face, being careful to avoid your eyes, and give yourself a few moments to lie back while the mask draws out puffiness and nourishes your skin. Rinse with warm water and follow with a toner.

As an extra bonus, cut up a second peach and pour a small amount of cream on top. Instead of rubbing this on your face, put it in your face! Enjoy a delightful, nutritious breakfast. Nourish the inside and the outside of your body!

Trust Your Instincts

Trusting our intuition often saves us from disaster.
—ANNE WILSON SCHAEF,
Meditations for Women Who Do Too Much (1990)

I'm fairly observant. In fact, minutes before a man robbed me at gunpoint, I noticed him loitering in front of my building. At the time I thought, "I'll bet he's up to no good. I'll call the police as soon as I get into the house." I never made it inside.

Learn from my mistake. If you see someone who looks suspicious, treat him with suspicion. Look at him, letting him know you registered his presence. Drive off. Get help. Don't do what I did and merely muse about your suspicions while giving an assailant the chance to pounce. Take your instincts seriously.

Embody Your Grief

If we have experienced a traumatic loss or many losses, we will have
a tendency to avoid pain by not allowing ourselves
to be connected to another person.
—CAROL C. WELL, *Right-Brain Sex* (1989)

As I sat sobbing in my therapist's office after my last romantic breakup, he beamed at me and said, "Well, you are so much healthier now! You didn't used to be able to care this deeply, and now you are grieving with your whole self." (Thanks a lot.)

I guess this is the good news-bad news about becoming more connected to your body. The pleasures are sweeter, and the pain is more potent. Since I've become more aware of my bodyself, I've noticed that I grieve losses not only on an emotional or intellectual level, but also at a body level. I physically crave the sound of his voice, the feel of his skin, the sight of his smile.

Losses may cause us to want to turn away from making peace with our bodies. We may try to protect ourselves from grief by separating ourselves, once again, from our senses, our appetites, our desire. As you deal with life's losses, no matter what form they may take, I urge you to stay connected to your body throughout the process, even though at times it may seem too painful. Pace yourself, but hold onto yourself. Once the pain subsides, there will be opportunity for deeper intimacy and more passionate pleasure. Don't lose hope. Don't let go of yourself.

Breathe Like a Choo-Choo Train

Breath is the junction point between mind, body, and spirit. Every change of mental state is reflected in the breath and then in the body.
—DEEPAK CHOPRA, M.D., *Ageless Body, Timeless Mind* (1993)

The little kid in you will enjoy this quick rejuvenator. Sit on the floor with your bottom touching the ground in-between your heels. Sit up straight and then blow out forcefully enough to make a "choo" noise. You'll need to pull your abdomen in quickly with each exhale to create enough intensity. Then repeat. Don't worry about the inhale. Believe me, that will take care of itself.

"Choo-choo" about ten times. Stop if you feel light-headed. Pretend to be a train in some exotic location—maybe the wild West, traveling through the Swiss Alps or along the Orient Express. When your train returns to town, your body will be relaxed, your cells oxygenated, and your mind alert and ready to go on your next adventure!

Confront Mortality

In youth it is easier (at least for some) to turn away from the facts of our infinitude, to pretend that they are unimportant. When we grow older, it becomes difficult to keep up the pretense.
—VALERIE C. SAIVING, "Our Body/Our Selves: Reflections on Sickness, Aging and Death" in *Journal of Feminist Studies in Religion*

Sometimes I wish I were all-powerful and able to accomplish any goal. Coming up against my limitations destroys this pretense. Often I experience my limitations via my body. Rather than deal with the painful reality of being finite and mortal, I find it easier to get angry at my body as if something horrible and unreasonable is being done to me.

It's easier to overcommit myself and then get angry at my body for needing rest than it is to say, "I'm sorry, but I can't take that project on right now." It's easier to complain about my defective brain during a migraine than it is to lower the stress in my life. Rather than accepting the natural aging process, I take the more convenient route of blaming my skin for wrinkling or my stomach for no longer enjoying green salsa or my hair for losing its color. The problem is not with my body but with my attitude about my limitations and the inevitability of death.

Are you blaming your body rather than accepting your limitations? Your limitations can teach you a great deal about life and death. Bring out your body journal. Select one of your physical limitations. Ask your limitation to share insights with you. Record a dialogue between yourself and your limitation. Make peace with mortality by accepting, at a deeper, spiritual level, the genuine limitations you experience in daily life.

Be Honest about Your Stress Level

Diminished well being is the social Pac-Man that devours coping and psychic energy and inner strength.
—BARBARA B. BROWN, *Between Health and Illness* (1984)

Write in the numbers indicating how often, if ever, the statements are true. Modify those statements that don't apply to you. 1—Never, 2—Sometimes, 3—Always.

___I set reasonable goals for myself.

___I function at a calm yet energized pace.

___I am early or arrive to appointments on time.

___I have an emotionally and financially rewarding work life.

___I have a nurturing and satisfying personal life.

___I pray daily letting go of what I cannot control.

___I look forward to something fun and/or nurturing every day.

___I drink one or less caffeinated drink per day.

___I exercise at least three times a week.

___I fall asleep and wake up relatively easily.

___I have a satisfying sex life.

___I listen when my body tells me I'm under too much stress.

___I ask for help when I need it.

___I schedule personal retreats and vacations on a regular basis.

___I receive massage regularly to assist in dealing with stress.

Scoring Evaluation

37-45   Congratulations! You're coping well with life's stresses.

26-36   Watch out. You're showing signs of stress distress.

0-25   Body alert! You may be at risk of stress-related illnesses.

Transform a Bad Habit

*Bad habits are trying to call our attention to some part of our lives
that is unlived or unexpressed.*
—SIDRA STONE

I have oodles of bad habits, and when I look at them closely,
many of them are not such terrible, sinister creatures. Most of
my bad habits are good intentions gone awry. For example, I want
to be a responsible, reliable person, so I work hard. Then I lose
control and commit myself to doing too much in too little time.
For extra energy, I motivate myself with anxiety, which triggers bursts
of adrenaline pouring into my bloodstream. Because I'm pumped
up, I can't sleep at night. I lose my appetite, I get sick and then I let
people down. Now, that's a bad habit. It started out well, but it
went haywire along the way.

Do you have any habits like this? What good intention lies
beneath it? Put energy into doing that good thing, so long as it's
reasonable, and commit yourself to discarding the self-destructive
pattern that wastes your time and undermines your health.

Celebrate Your Tears

[J]ust as the moving waters preceded the appearance of the rainbow in the primeval light, so does weeping precede the rainbow of illuminating light in the soul.
—VALENTIN TOMBERG, *Covenant of the Heart* (1994)

Typically, it is more acceptable for women in this culture to cry than it is for men, but even so, I'd rather not cry at all. I don't like to cry by myself and I especially hate crying in front of anyone else. In fact, some friends I've known for years have never seen me cry. Only in a few situations do I let the tears flow.

If you are like me in this regard, then neither of us is taking advantage of our bodies' attempt to help us feel better. Not only do tears offer us an emotional release, but studies have shown that tears release endorphins, one of the body's pain relievers. Some researchers also believe that tears cleanse the body of wastes, hormones, and other potentially harmful substances. So, the next time you feel those tears welling up, don't hold them back. Whether you cry in public or in private, let the tears flow. You and your body will feel better.

Let Out Frustration

For millions of people, life is so frustrating that their only hope of relieving stress is by overeating and drinking, while whole societies try to escape their miseries by attacking other countries. Strife breaks out over issues that seem trivial to an outsider, but frustration and lack of control are enormously painful conditions to live under.
—DEEPAK CHOPRA, M.D., *Ageless Body, Timeless Mind* (1993)

Frustration is more than emotion. It's a physiological condition that can make you vulnerable to disease, premature aging, and even death. Recognizing that pent-up frustration is life-threatening is the first step. The second step is *doing* something with it.

We're most often frustrated by situations over which we have no control. Even innocuous situations, such as misplacing one's keys, can result in intense frustration. We need the keys but can't find the keys. The helplessness can agitate us into a fury.

When you're frustrated, ask yourself if your goal is genuinely important. If you want to do an errand that can be done later, release the goal and hope that the keys will turn up later. But if you need to drive to work, channel your frustration into regaining control, for example, by asking others to search for the keys or by digging up a spare set. Use your frustration as energy for coping and problem-solving.

Even if you've handled frustration effectively, usually some stress lingers after the situation is resolved. Find a release, such as playing racquetball, recording your feelings in your body journal, dancing around the living room, or throwing the keys on the floor once you find them. Select a genuinely satisfying activity that has no negative consequences for you or anyone else.

Parent Yourself

*To some extent, we all make parents of our partners. . . . When
partners establish too strong a parent-child relationship, it evokes the
incest taboo, shutting down sexual response.*
—CAROL C. WELL, *Right-Brain Sex* (1989)

Since none of us were raised by perfect parents, we all have some
unfinished childhood business to conduct. Most often, we take
this business into our romantic relationships, unconsciously asking
our mates to father or mother us. I believe this dynamic is
unavoidable, and need not pose a substantial threat to your
relationship. If, however, your need to be a child in your romantic
relationship outweighs your ability to be an adult, your physical
relationship will be adversely affected. Most often this takes the
form of decreased sexual interest and response, since parent-child
relating will evoke the incest taboo.

Do you look to your mate to satisfy unmet childhood needs? Do
you want the nurturance of a mother or the protection of a father?
How does this affect your body's response?

Or maybe the roles are reversed and you feel like your partner
has put you in the mothering role. Does this dynamic attract you
sexually or leave you feeling maternal, but turned off?

Pay attention to the way your body responds to your partner to
assess whether or not either or both of you are trying to get childhood needs met in an inappropriate way. Take responsibility for
addressing your unfinished childhood issues. This may entail getting
into a support group, seeing a therapist, doing inner child work, or
participating in body work. Rather than expect your partner to
parent you, look outside your romantic relationship for the help
you need and deserve.

Think of Health, Honor, and Comfort

Resolve to think of nothing but . . . health in the first place and . . .
honor and comfort in the second, because in this fickle world
we can do nothing else, and those who do not know how
to spend their time profitably allow their lives to slip away
with much sorrow and little praise.
—ISABELLE D'ESTE (1474-1530), in RACHEL ERLANGER,
Lucrezia Borgia (1978)

Even though Isabelle d'Este lived nearly five centuries ago, she understood the importance of self-care, not merely from a short-sighted perspective but from evaluating how best we can all use the time God gives us.

In your body journal, first describe one healthy action you have taken in the last week to strengthen your immune system. Did you exercise? Tell a friend you were angry rather than hold it in? Laugh with a loved one?

Second, describe something you have done in the last week that honored your body. Maybe you took twenty minutes to relax in a warm bath. Or you may have noticed a knot in your stomach and steered clear of a hostile co-worker. Maybe you felt a headache coming on and instead of getting frustrated with yourself, you took a short nap and woke up refreshed.

Third, describe a way you comforted yourself in the past week. Did you get a soothing massage? Take a leisurely walk while listening to the birds? Did you curl up in the arms of your partner to receive the joys of emotional and physical affection?

Acknowledge your progress in past weeks.

Honor the Earth

The maltreatment of the natural world and its impoverishment leads to the impoverishment of the human soul.
—Raisa M. Gorbachev, *I Hope* (1991)

I recently decided to become a vegetarian for several reasons. First, the more I care about my health, the more selective I am about food. Nutritionists urge us to eat more fresh fruits and vegetables and less fat and meat products. A second reason is my growing concern for the environment. For example, rain forests are destroyed so that more beef can be raised. Third, eating meat is no longer attractive to me when I acknowledge animal suffering.

When I trade a possessive view of the earth for a sense of responsibility, my eyes open to new possibilities and pain. I grieve the ways I've contributed to pollution, the destruction of animal life, and the disregard of future generations. Out of this sadness comes a resolve to contribute to the healing between myself and the planet upon which I live.

Join me in this endeavor. While becoming a vegetarian may not be for you, find one way that you can contribute to the earth today, a path that you've never walked before. If you don't recycle your cans and plastic goods, start today. If you use detergents that are hostile to the environment, discard them safely and purchase biodegradable soaps and cleaners. Contribute to a local animal reserve. Contact your city hall for information about tree-planting projects in your area. Take one step, any step, toward making peace with the earth and consequently, peace with yourself.

Be Young

*One remains young as long as one can still learn, can still take on
new habits, can bear contradictions.*
—Marie von Ebner-Eschenbach (1830-1916)

Are you remaining young regardless of your chronological age?
Nicholas, the six-month-old son of close friends, has recently
reminded me to try fresh approaches to old problems. Just at the
crawling age, Nicholas has developed his own method for getting
across the room. Rather than crawl on his stomach, he lies flat on
his back. Then he arches his back, pulls his feet in, and pushes
himself forward. He can zip across the room like a little inchworm.

Nicholas created a unique solution to an age-old transportation
question. Try a new approach to one of your problems. Instead of
relying on medication to fall asleep at night, try an herbal remedy
for insomnia or drink warm milk right before retiring. Rather than
reach for an aspirin bottle to ease a nagging headache, try applying
warm or cold compresses to the back of your neck. Maybe drinking
a large amount of water will help. Experiment with the enthusiasm
of a youngster. And of course, if a problem persists contact your
doctor.

Be young today. Respond to an old question with a new answer
by using your body's wisdom in a way you've never tried.

Locate Sadness in Your Body

Sorrow was like the wind. It came in gusts, shaking the woman.
She braced herself.
—MARJORIE KINNAN RAWLINGS, *South Moon Under* (1933)

I remember clumsily groping for the ringing phone in the early morning darkness. The news that my uncle had died in a car accident shot through my ear and ricocheted through my body. Even though I wasn't fully awake, my body tightened in sadness.

Our bodies express sadness in many ways. Crying is perhaps the mode of expression we most commonly associate with grief. But tears are but one way sorrow inhabits our bodies. Shallow breathing, lack of energy, and slumped shoulders also let us know that we are sorrowful. Sadness can be quietly held in the body, or feel like a bolt of lightening shattering our sense of predictability. In body work sessions, my clients and I have discovered sadness in all parts of the body—knotted along the spine, clenched in the palm of the hand, or buried in the center of the calf.

How does your body share your sadness? Locate feelings of sorrow in your body. Record your insights in your body journal to help you better understand yourself, your body, and your pain. To resolve your sadness, share your feelings with your body buddy or someone else you love.

Celebrate Your Nose Hairs

*Besides smelling, warming, and humidifying inhaled air, another
important function performed by the nose is defense against airborne
bacteria. A constant flow of mucus and the movement of tiny
hairlike cilia carry bacteria to the back of the throat, where they
drain into the stomach—and are vanquished by the digestive acids.*
—CARL KOCH AND JOYCE HEIL, *Created in God's Image* (1991)

Okay, how often do you express gratitude to your nose hairs? I
suspect not very often. But I think nose hairs get a bum rap.
Think about what they do for us. Those tiny hairs filter out dust,
lint, and flying bugs that don't belong in our lungs. Plus, those tiny
particles that sneak inside are moved slowly out of our nostrils by
our nose hairs. They help our sinuses work well and aid our immune
system when we become ill.

Celebrate your nose hairs and all the fresh air they allow into
your lungs by giving your nose a gentle blow of gratitude. Thank
your hairs for all they do to keep you breathing and keep you healthy.

Be a Lie Detector

Most of us sense what feels safe and what doesn't. We intuit who's
trustworthy and who's feeding us a line. But as time passes
we forget. We train ourselves to disregard the early cues,
to be ever so reasonable, to be relentlessly polite.
—DORY HOLLANDER, *101 Lies Men Tell Women* (1995)

I remember calling the man I was dating at his home and hearing a woman's voice answer the phone. She said she was just a friend, but my stomach flipped over and my throat constricted. Somehow I just knew there was more going on.

When I asked him about her, he dismissed my concern as unjustified jealousy. Only after our relationship ended did I discover that they were indeed involved and their relationship contributed a great deal to our break-up.

How did I know? My body told me. My ears told me by the odd tone in his voice as he denied misconduct. Tightness in my stomach told me not to trust his words. But I wanted to trust him more than myself. At the time, I thought trusting myself would cost me too much—a man I loved.

I lost the relationship anyway, along with my sense of dignity for believing his lies. If I had listened to my body I would have had to face inevitable losses, but I would have kept faith with myself.

Is someone in your life telling you things that contradict what your body is saying? Think before you dismiss the dryness in your mouth, the sweat between your shoulder blades, or the fact that you're holding your breath. Follow your body's wisdom. You'll suffer less in the long run.

Learn from Women Who Know

This is life. Your life. . . . Are you getting what you need?
Are you loving and caring for yourself? And if not, why not?
—JENNIFER LOUDEN, *The Woman's Comfort Book* (1992)

I grew up watching my parents use art supplies to paint, draw, and create items of beauty. Simply by being around people who knew how to use art supplies I developed a working knowledge of how to choose appropriate tools to express myself artistically.

Those who were not exposed to such tools may be hard-pressed to tell a brush for watercolors from one best suited for oil. We often learn by observing others, and if we haven't had models for a particular skill, it is unlikely that we'll have mastered those skills.

One reason many of us don't take better care of ourselves is simply that we do not know how. Few of us have had the chance to observe women who are skilled in the art of self-care. Look around and notice the women in your life, whether close by or less-known, who demonstrate a healthy, self-nurturing love. Approach one of them, asking her how she takes care of her body. Find out the ingredients for a cucumber-milk face mask or the phone number of a nurturing massage therapist or the date of the next dance class at the city college. Record this new information in your body journal. Women who take care of themselves know important skills that they can teach and that you can learn.

Set Up a Drinking Plan

It's all right to drink like a fish if you drink what a fish drinks.
—MARY PETTIBONE POOLE

Remember the ad for beer that claimed, "It's the water?" We can apply that same statement to our bodies. What keeps our blood flowing, our lymph system healthy, our muscles strong and flexible, our organs vital, our taste buds tasting, and our brains secure in our skulls? It's the water.

Drink a lot of water every day. I keep on my desk a drinking bottle that holds one liter of water. My goal is to drink two of these each day. I've found that if the water is there, easy to reach, I'm more likely to drink the amount of water I need. Also, having water handy tends to keep me from craving less-healthy drinks such as soda or coffee.

Set up a drinking plan for yourself that is easy and works for you. Nurture yourself from the inside out with lots of fresh, delicious water.

Sense Your Senses

[W]hat is beyond our senses we cannot know.
—DIANE ACKERMAN, *A Natural History of the Senses* (1990)

W*hat should I wear?*

That's a question we ask ourselves each morning as we look groggy-eyed at the clothes in our closets. Rather than make this decision from a solely pragmatic point of view, bring your senses into the conversation. Let your sensual desires help you decide. When selecting a power outfit appropriate for your profession, factor in how wonderful a particular fabric feels against your skin or the visual pleasure you take in wearing a favorite color. Select a sweater that is particularly soft or earrings that tickle your neck as they swing from your ear lobes. Include your body more actively in your decision-making process, paying special attention to the joy gained through your senses.

Enjoy Spring

I love spring anywhere, but if I could choose
I would always greet it in a garden.
—RUTH STOUT, *How to Have a Green Thumb*
Without an Aching Back (1955)

Every spring I buy new herbs for my kitchen window box. This year I grew oregano, which I dried and used on pasta (that's about as gourmet as my cooking gets). I also had several fresh basil plants. I sliced fresh tomatoes, covered each slice with fresh basil leaves, sprinkled on olive oil spiced with a bit of my oregano, and munched to my heart's delight.

Winter is subsiding and spring is beginning to push her way into our world. Pick up an herb plant or two and herald the beginning of spring, a time of growth and rebirth. Enjoy this spring season by treating your taste buds to the joys of herbs.

Pay Attention

Suppress everything in the child.
—DANIEL GOTTLIEB MORITZ SCHREBER,
in JULES OLDER, *Touching is Healing* (1982)

B *e quiet. All you want is attention!*
Daniel Schreber, a respected German doctor and educator, led a crusade around the turn of the century for parents to control, if not squelch, the emotions of their children. Mothers were warned not to treat their children with "gentleness," especially if all they wanted was attention, because they'd develop the emotion of "spite."

Sadly, this attitude dominated child-rearing ideas well into the twentieth century, most likely impacting how you and I were treated as children. If we were hungry or our diapers were wet, those were *real* needs, and parents were expected to respond. But if all we wanted was attention, well, that wasn't a real need, and parents were instructed to refuse to respond. We may now believe that our needs for attention are legitimate, but without meaning to, treat ourselves with the same disrespect propagated by past generations. Do you discredit your own needs by saying to yourself, "Oh, stop it! All you want is attention"?

Take time to relax for a moment and ask yourself, "What sort of attention do I need today?" Does your skin need nurturing? How about treating yourself to a facial? Maybe your feet are aching and would love a soothing foot massage. Is there tension between your shoulder blades? Fifteen minutes of stretching and breathing exercises may be just what you need. Weary after a busy, noisy day? A few minutes resting while listening to a favorite CD may transform you. Pay attention to yourself. Getting attention is a legitimate need.

MAY

OAK TREES

Silhouette sticks.
Sometimes frosted or heavy with wet white.
Otherwise shockingly bare profiles
against the winter sky.

Green life suddenly exploding
out of dead wood.
Resurrection miracles.
Proclaimers of better days to come.

Full leafed shade-makers.
Taken-for-granted protectors.
Stately, beloved observers
of summer fun.

Red-orange blazes.
Breath-catching announcers of change.
Raining bright colors
in a whirling dance with the wind.

Rooted. Faithful to what
they were created to be.
Oak trees only and completely.
Reflecting a unique part of the Creator's joy.

Wise friends.
Teaching me the basic truth
of the beauty of being.
Reminding me to be me.

Live Sensuously

It's that interchange between the embodied soul and the outside
world that is the dynamic process. That's how growth takes place.
That is life.
—MARION WOODMAN, *Conscious Femininity* (1995)

Although I go out to dinner regularly with my two friends, Joel and Pat, it can be a challenge agreeing on a restaurant. Joel is an artistic man who likes to go to trendy, well decorated restaurants. I resist because these restaurants rarely have carpeting on the floors and usually place tables close together. Since the joy of sharing dinner for me is the conversation, I want to go somewhere quiet so we can talk. Pat usually stares at us in amazement as our debate never mentions the food. Dinner, to Pat, is a culinary experience. She can't imagine choosing a place to eat on any basis other than the taste of the food.

The three of us demonstrate how our senses influence our individual experience. While we can receive nourishment through all of our senses, most of us have a dominant sense through which we enjoy life—a visual style, a kinesthetic or "body" style, or an auditory style. Let's say you were asked to describe your winter vacation. If you are a visual person, you will have a tendency to describe how your vacation looked, perhaps using words such as *bright, colorful, dark, clear,* or *vague.* For example, you might say, "The view from the chalet was postcard-perfect, with the snow white and glistening as far as the eye could see."

If you have a body style, however, you would be more likely to describe how your experience felt, "A cold wind blew up in the late afternoon. It was hard to ski because the snow iced up in patches, making it extremely slippery. It sure felt good to get back to the chalet, where we warmed by the fire and sipped hot cider."

If you're an auditory person, like me, you would probably describe how your vacation sounded, using words such as *quiet, harmonious, musical,* or *thundering.* You might say, "What struck me most was how quiet it was on the slopes with the snow dampening every sound. As I rode the lift, all I heard was the faint, squeaking gears against the cables and the skiers swishing below. Everything was so quiet at the top, all I could hear was my heart pounding with excitement."

What impressed you about your last vacation? The vivid sunset? Your children's smiles? If so, maybe you're a visual person. Or do you most remember the taste of the cuisine? The warmth of your partner's body by your side? If you are most connected to sensations, you may have a body style. Perhaps you remember the calypso music as it floated over the lagoon or the laughter of your travel companions. Are the conversations you had still ringing in your ears? You may have an auditory style.

Find your own style. Do something pleasing today for your particular dominant sense.

Assess Your Stress

The Amish love the Sunshine and Shadow quilt pattern. It shows
two sides—the dark and light, spirit and form—and the challenge
of bringing the two into a larger unity. It's not a choice between
extremes. . . . It's a balancing act that includes opposites.
—SUE BENDER, *Plain and Simple* (1989)

Are you living in harmony with your body? Are you getting an adequate amount of rest while being challenged by creative activity? Is there a balance between your "down" time and the various demands on your energy and attention? Are you getting as much as you give?

If you are out of balance, your body will register stress in your muscles, your organs, your nervous system. Pull out your body journal and assess your stress level this month.

Draw an outline of your body and color in the stressed-out places. Your shoulders may be so tight they're up around your ears. The back of your calves may be sore and cramping. Your lungs may have trouble breathing because you're carrying so much stress in your abdomen. Mark it all down.

Compare this drawing with past renditions. What can you learn about the stress levels in your life? How is stress affecting your body? Are there changes you need to make in order to restore balance in your life? Talk these questions over with your body buddy or someone else you feel understands.

Honor Others' Boundaries

Boundaries are really about relationship, and finally about love.
—HENRY CLOUD AND JOHN TOWNSEND, *Boundaries* (1992)

Most of us want to see ourselves as good people—kind and loving women who contribute positively to those around us. However, the truth is that if we disregard our own bodies, we will unwittingly disregard the bodies of those we care about.

One way I've hurt others is by unintentionally violating their boundaries because I was unclear about where my personal space ended and theirs began. I often got "too close for comfort" or gave the impression I didn't care by standing back too far. Skilled in ignoring the signals my body gave me, I was quite adept at ignoring the body signals others gave me as well.

It is a sobering, but helpful exercise to ask your close friends and family members how you have violated their boundaries. Perhaps physically, by getting into their space. Or emotionally, by saying something hurtful or degrading about their bodies. Maybe you pushed someone too hard or didn't give the support they needed because you didn't acknowledge their physical or emotional limitations. Ask and see. And if you have hurt someone else, ask that person one more question, "How can I make amends?"

Learn from the Animals

There are people who live lives little different than the beasts, and I don't mean that badly. I mean that they accept whatever happens day to day without struggle or question or regret. To them things just are, like the earth and sky and seasons.
—CELESTE DE BLASIS, *Wild Swan* (1984)

Recently I took a break from writing and walked downstairs to see my two cats, Sassy and Stud, stretched out on their backs, legs strewn unceremoniously apart, heads back, thoroughly enjoying an afternoon nap. At the sound of my approach, Sassy woke up, looked at me out of one yellow eye, and curled around in the most delicious stretch I've ever witnessed. Stud continued his snooze, undaunted. These two are great examples of embodied pleasure.

Take some time today and observe your pet or the pet of a friend. If you have no pets, you may want to visit the zoo. Pick an animal, and watch how that animal unabashedly lives in his or her body. No apology. Just sheer enjoyment of being alive. If you are at home, get down on the floor and follow their movement. Shake your body with glee along with your dog or snuggle like your cat. We have a lot to learn from animals about living in our bodies. Take time for a lesson today.

Be Big

Women should try to increase their size rather than decrease it,
because I believe the bigger we are, the more space we'll take up, and
the more we'll have to be reckoned with.
—ROSEANNE, Comedian

I remember playing softball as a child and hearing the boys complain about having girls on their team. "They can't throw a ball worth a darn," I heard one say. Another mimicked the way most of us girls threw balls, triggering chuckles from the other boys.

Why is it that girls have in the past been less adept at sports? One reason is that in order to properly throw a ball or execute other athletic maneuvers, one has to move the body in such a way as to take up a lot of space. Legs need to be apart to provide a solid base, the torso must be free to swing, and the shoulders should be up and open, with arms outstretched and moving. One has to feel comfortable taking up space to throw a ball correctly.

Traditionally, girls were taught to be "small," to sit with their legs crossed while boys took up more space with their legs apart. Girls were to walk along a dainty imaginary line while boys were allotted more space in which to strut, swagger, or stride. Girls' sense of smallness carried over to sports where we were reluctant to take up space. Instead, we tended to throw with one arm, shoulders down, with insufficient support from our legs, held close together.

Claim the space you and your body need today. Be big, be wide, be tall. Swing your arms, sway your torso, let your feet go anywhere they want. Be a force to be reckoned with.

Decorate Yourself

Lots of women buy just as many wigs and makeup things as I do.
They just don't wear them all at the same time.
—DOLLY PARTON, in BARBARA MCDOWELL AND HANA UMLAUF,
Women's Almanac (1977)

Why should any of us be slaves to fashion? I say: Be your own woman! If you want to wear false eyelashes, blond wigs, and stiletto heels, go for it. If sneakers and old blue jeans make you happy, then enjoy your casual style. Some women love lace and flowers. Others love sleek, bold colors and accessorize with black.

However you decorate your body, enjoy yourself. And like Dolly, don't take it too seriously. Your body is beautiful, without all the baubles and bangles and bows. So have fun with clothes. They are just not that important, after all.

Locate Happiness in Your Body

Birds sing after a storm; why shouldn't people
feel as free to delight in whatever remains to them?
—ROSE KENNEDY, *Times to Remember* (1974)

My friend's voice bounced from the phone receiver like a beach ball on a windy day. "I got the job! Can you believe it? All this work has finally paid off!"

We were both thrilled at her accomplishment, laughing and chatting together for another hour or so. Happiness is an emotion that often shows itself in our voices. Like a raucous wave splashing over the beach and erasing a sand castle, happiness bursts through our voices, replacing tired tones with a giggle and a lilt.

How does your body express happiness? Through the smile on your face? A wiggle in your walk? A deep and long-needed sigh? Can you let yourself whoop and jump up and down? Locate happiness in your body and record your findings in your body journal. Then share your happiness with a friend!

Rub Yourself the Right Way

It isn't the great big pleasures that count the most;
it's making a great deal out of the little ones.
—JEAN WEBSTER, *Daddy-Long-Legs* (1912)

When I'm especially busy, my body is under additional stress and needs more care than when I'm living life calmly. My body needs more from me because I'm asking more from my body. But here's the rub—I'm too busy to give extra attention to my body when my body needs nurturance the most.

If I view taking care of myself as yet another major obligation, then my body gets neglected during the busy times in my life. But if I see body-care as something I can do quickly and easily, finding a few minutes somewhere in a demanding day is possible.

Sit comfortably on the floor with your shoes off. If you are wearing panty hose, that's fine. This foot rub works great regardless.

Pull one foot towards you, sole down, and gently massage and rotate each toe. Take your time. These little guys work hard for you, often scrunched up in ill-fitting shoes.

Next, place your thumbs side-by-side on the top of your foot, with your fingers meeting underneath. Gently pull your feet out to either side, stretching the bones in your foot away from each other. Repeat several times.

Lastly, with your finger tips, rub small circles around your ankles. Some believe massaging the foot stimulates the entire body. You'll emerge from this short rub feeling rejuvenated, grounded, and more at home with your whole body.

Don't Second-Guess Yourself

Most women aren't exactly sure of their boundaries.
They don't know when to say yes or no or to assert themselves.
—PAXTON QUIGLEY, *Not An Easy Target* (1995)

My cats have taught me a lot about boundaries. Both Sassy and Stud are very clear about their "space." The other day, a neighbor's cat ran into our living room and headed straight for the food bowls. Both cats were clear that they did not want this newcomer in their area, eating their food. Without hesitation, tails puffed out, hair along their spines raised, and hissing filled the air. A boundary had been crossed, and it was defended with feline fervor.

I'm not always sure when my boundaries are crossed. If I'm paying attention to my body, I feel my jaw tighten or a tingle go up my spine or a quick gasp for breath. But unlike my cats, I worry: Will I hurt someone else's feelings? Have I misinterpreted the situation? Will I be seen as too pushy or overly emotional? And all the while I'm wandering through this maze of second-guesses, someone is violating my space.

None of us perfectly assesses each and every situation. So, accepting the fact that we all err, choose to err on the side of your boundaries. Trust that tightening in your throat, that intuition of danger, that twitching of your eyelid. Set your boundary, and if it turns out you overreacted, that's okay. Just ask my cats.

Sense Love All around You

In the end, nothing we do or say in this lifetime will matter
as much as the way we have loved one another.
—DAPHNE ROSE KINGMA, *True Love* (1991)

What convinces you that someone loves you? Do you communicate and receive love through one of three sensory channels: visual, auditory, or kinesthetic?

Visual people feel loved by demonstrations they can see, such as receiving a beautiful card or sharing a gorgeous sunset with someone special. Those who, like myself, are auditory need to hear affectionate words spoken to feel truly loved. Kinesthetic or body people have to literally feel love through touch. Love is received through a warm hug, a gentle caress, or a passionate kiss.

Take time to notice how you feel love. Ask your mate or loved ones to give you affection through the means you receive love best. Then ask your mate or other loved ones how they best receive your affection. Make an effort to give to them in ways that nurture them, rather than simply giving what feels best to you. Share love effectively, using sensory channels. It will enhance your love life significantly.

Denounce Deprivation

This is what I have seen to be good: it is fitting to eat and drink and find enjoyment in all toil with which one toils under the sun for the few days of life God gives us; for this is our lot.
—ECCLESIASTES 5:18, *New Revised Standard Version*

My therapist looked at me with alarm when I told her I was using a laxative. She told me in no uncertain terms that if I didn't eat more and put on weight, she would put me in the hospital for an eating disorder. At the time, I thought she was out of her mind. I didn't have an eating disorder. I just didn't eat anything, that's all.

Denying the severity of the problem is a symptom of someone who is actively engaged in an addictive eating disorder. Sufferers of anorexia nervosa or other forms of compulsive food-depriving behavior feel they must continually lose weight to achieve a sense of peace or well-being. The sense of emptiness becomes so familiar that any form of nurturance may feel uncomfortable or even intolerable. Back then, my thinking was so distorted that I secretly congratulated myself on how little I had eaten on a particular day.

Do you feel proud of yourself when you deprive your body of what you need? If you are like I was, depriving your body of food may be your temptation. But you may deprive yourself of other things, such as rest, exercise, compliments, quality health care, or simply acceptance. Locate one area in which you deprive yourself and turn the tide. Give to yourself the nurturance you deserve.

Embody Spirituality

That which affects the life of the body affects the life of the soul;
in the same way, without the soul as its source of life,
the body has no life of its own.
—RAY S. ANDERSON, *Self Care* (1995)

I used to have an invisible dotted line across my neck dividing the good (my mind and pure thoughts) from all that was bad (my body, sexual desires, and my emotions). Cutting myself up into pieces, such as "head," "heart," "body," and "soul," led to assigning rank to each piece. The mind had higher status than the heart, the soul was precious while the body was unimportant.

My journey has led me toward *embodied spirituality*, viewing both the seen (the body) and the unseen (the soul) as vital to a living, growing spiritual self. Worshipping the body alone or valuing the soul above all deprives us of full, vibrant spirituality.

Take out your body journal and write down your reflections on these questions:

♦ Define the term "spirit."

♦ Define the term "body."

♦ How do these aspects of self relate to one another?

♦ Do you adhere to a spiritual perspective that elevates one part over the other? If yes, please describe. (For example, do you practice meditation that suggests spiritual enlightenment is found by transcending the body? Have you been taught that your body is not to be trusted and must be controlled?)

♦ What changes need to be made in your spiritual understanding that would bring reconciliation between your body and spirit?

Start implementing those changes and make room in your spirituality for all parts of you.

Love Where You Are

The most mundane building can be transformed through the spirit
with which it is used, expressed in the flower in the window, the
well-scrubbed doorstep, or the smell of freshly baked bread.
—THOMAS BENDER, *The Power of Place*

Moving into my condo, I was thrilled with the additional space it afforded in comparison to the small apartment I had just left. But as my friends moved to even larger homes, my place gradually seemed cramped and inferior.

How does one make a home in which contentment can live? Certainly not by living according to a motto of "Bigger, stronger, newer. More, more, more." The square footage or a name on the deed doesn't make a home. A home is created when love makes a place for the body to rest, to eat, to touch, to laugh, to enjoy daily living.

The more "body friendly" I make my place, the more content I am with where I live. I enjoy the quiet of my home, the comfort of my soft couch, and the photographs of friends framed on my walls. The more I attend to my home's sensual comforts, the more this place made of wood and plaster becomes a source of nurturance, protection, and renewal.

Are you content with the space in which you live? Make it "body friendly," using your sensory style. If you're visual, plant some colorful flowers or display a painting you've created. If you're kinesthetic, make some soft pillows for the floor, or juice some fresh oranges. If you're auditory, get that CD you've been wanting, or invite a friend over for an evening of conversation. Love will transform even the simplest place into a home.

Be Happy, Be Beautiful

A mode of conduct, a standard of courage, discipline, fortitude, and integrity can do a great deal to make a woman beautiful.
—JACQUELINE BISSET, in *The Los Angeles Times* (1974)

Of the many things I've been surprised to learn as a massage therapist is that many of us carry a lot of stress in our scalps. The more I've thought about it, though, the more sense it makes, because we often make faces when we're unhappy or stressed.

Look around and you'll see tension in other people's faces: pinched lines between people's eyebrows, clenched jaws, a deep frown. Each time we scrunch up our faces, we add a little stress to the muscles in our scalp.

Now look around and find someone who appears calm and happy. Eyes are open and relaxed, and lips are soft and smile easily. A happy face appears fuller, healthier, and younger. Conducting ourselves with courage, and seeking serenity and happiness contributes a great deal to our beauty. Loving yourself will do more for your appearance than all the creams and concoctions you'll ever apply to your skin.

Celebrate Your Face

It is said that the face is the mirror of the soul.
—ROSWITHA OF GANDERSHEIM (935-1000), *The Plays of Roswitha*,
CHRISTOPHER ST. JOHN, TR. (1923)

I looked into the vibrating mirror in the airplane restroom and saw the return stare of a woman with puffy, bloodshot eyes and a sour disposition. The combination of dry air in the plane cabin and the length of my flight had left my sinuses arid, my skin drawn, and my eyes unhappy.

After wiping the sink clean, I filled it with the coldest water I could stand and soaked my hands for a few moments. The cold caused me to take a quick breath, which reminded me that I hadn't been breathing very deeply. After my hands were cold, I placed them on my face over my eyes. The cold was so soothing.

Once my hands had warmed, I began to gently massage my forehead, temples, jaw (a tender spot for me), and down to my chin. My face and my mood were much happier now.

Try this simple exercise whenever you feel sluggish or tired. Your face will feel cared for and your soul will be replenished.

Drive the Speed Limit

One hand full of rest is better than two fists full of labor
and striving after the wind.
—ECCLESIASTES 4:6, *New American Standard Bible*

Dashing between lanes, I was trying to make up time for starting out late. I didn't get to the meeting any earlier. In fact, I arrived even later because I was pulled over by a highway patrolman who didn't take kindly to my acting out my stress at seventy-five miles per hour.

It is impossible to live in an alert processing state if you're driving like a mad woman, darting in-between cars and swearing at other motorists under your breath. You cannot turn your car into an airplane. So you're late. Face it. Accept it.

And let your body relax into an alert processing state. Not only will you do your body a favor by lowering your stress level, you may also avoid getting into an accident due to impaired judgment or reckless driving. Be late. Be alive. Be healthy.

Get Some Mothering

I cannot forget my mother. Though not as sturdy as others, she is my bridge. When I needed to get across, she steadied herself long enough for me to run across safely.
—RENITA WEEMS, "Hush, Mama's Gotta Go Bye-Bye," in PATRICIA BELL-SCOTT ET AL., EDS., *Double Stitch* (1991)

I put my hands gently around the head of one of my clients, and tears began streaming down her face. When she felt ready to talk, she told me, "I always wanted my mother to hold me, touch me in a soft way, but she never did. I've tried to pretend I don't need anyone, just like she did. But when you touched my hair, all that longing came back to me."

Many women do not feel nurtured sufficiently by their mothers. A nurturing mother pays attention to the physical needs of her children. Are they eating nutritious meals, are they getting enough exercise and rest, are they receiving enough hugs? If our needs for touch, body acceptance, good nutrition, and exercise are ignored, then we can grow up longing for more.

Do you often long for some mothering attention? Think about how you can meet that need now. If your mother is no longer living or is unable to nurture you for other reasons, try finding another woman who is able and willing to give you some loving attention. You can help provide the mothering you need by paying attention to your body the way a loving mother would care for a child. There is still time to get what you need. Take advantage of the present opportunities for better mothering in your life.

Love Yourself through a Headache

Back in the Middle Ages, when people thought demons in the brain caused headaches, treatment consisted of boring a small hole in the skull. Fortunately, doctors understand headaches a little better today . . .
—DON R. POWELL, *365 Health Hints* (1990)

I hate headaches, and I get all three kinds: tension, sinus, and migraine. It's easy to blame my head for hurting, thinking things like, "Look, I don't have time to spend in bed with you throbbing all day." I've been known to clench my jaw and storm angrily toward the medicine cabinet in avowed war against my head. Of course, blaming my head for the pain is a waste of time. My frustration and increased tension merely intensify the pain and duration of the headache.

These days I'm working on a new approach. I view my head as the messenger and the pain as a message. Taking whatever medication is advised and then resting, I ask myself, "What is the message?"

Rarely is the message hard to figure out. For me, tension headaches usually mean I have too many deadlines to meet in too little time. Sinus headaches can be environmentally caused but are often intensified by diet, such as dairy products. Migraines may signal a letdown after a stressful situation concludes, providing the chance (whether I want it or not) to reflect on how to lower my stress.

Listen to the pain, and love yourself through the headache. You'll learn a lot more about how to prevent headaches in the future, and your head will be happier, too.

Sense Your Way to the Holy

Listen to your life. See it for the fathomless mystery that it is. In the
boredom and pain of it no less than in the excitement
and gladness: touch, taste, smell your way to the
holy and hidden heart of it because in the last analysis
all moments are key moments, and life itself is grace.
—FREDERICK BUECHNER, *Now and Then* (1983)

The first time I saw the Grand Canyon, it took my breath away:
the expanse, the depth, the blazing red rock. Peeking over the
steep banks, I seemed small and insignificant, and yet, at the same
time, a part of whatever the Grand Canyon was a part of—
something powerful, lasting, and wise. At that moment I was
convinced that God exists, although I can't articulate my conviction
to anyone else's satisfaction. And I feel no need to do so. There is
something inside my own body that heard God's whispering voice
in the wind whistling through the canyon walls.

How do you sense God's presence? Which of your senses draws
you closest to what is forever, what is good, what is complete? Do
you see God in the eyes of someone you love? Hear God's voice in
the steady patter of spring rain? Taste God's goodness when biting
into a fresh peach? Feel God's touch as ocean waves splash across
your feet? Smell God's power in the cold, clean air following a
snowfall? Taste, smell, see, touch, and hear God through the natural
displays of grace that exist all around you.

Be Spontaneous

If I claim one guiding principle for my life,
it is to say yes to unusual propositions and see what happens.
—BARBARA BROWN TAYLOR, *Women of the Word:*
Contemporary Sermons by Women Clergy (1985)

Ask any of my friends, and they will tell you I am not a spontaneous person. In fact, I tend to schedule my time at least nine months in advance. Doing something on the spur of the moment is quite uncharacteristic. But as I've been thinking about this quote from Barbara Brown Taylor, I've realized that my life would be richer, my body would be happier, and my friends would be relieved if I said "yes" to an unusual proposition and simply enjoyed the uncertainty of the path.

Take a look at your day-to-day traits and decide to involve your body in something out of the ordinary. Wear a color unusual for you. Taste a flavor you rarely try. Experiment with a new scent. Drive home along a different route. Call up a friend with whom you've lost touch. Follow a different path today, and see what happens. Enjoy the adventure!

Embrace Your Demons

Whatever we resist—persists. These demons, these parts of us that haunt us, torture us, and reduce us, are the agents of change. They throw down the gauntlet to the warrior within us to face them in a duel.

—STEPHANIE ERICSSON, *Companion Through the Darkness* (1993)

Although I had worked long hours writing the manuscript for this book, the deadline date approached, arrived, and zoomed past me like a speeding car. Not wanting to let down the folks at the publishing house, I worked even harder for longer hours, writing how important it is to honor your body, especially during times of stress. Too bad writing about it isn't enough.

My body finally insisted on some balance in my life by putting me in bed with a serious sinus infection. I smiled to myself as I pulled the covers up around my ears, finally compliant and willing to rest. What did my sinus infection teach me? It isn't enough to *know* about health. One has to *do* health. If I can learn from that insight, my body won't have to take extreme measures to make me rest.

I don't like having limitations. It seems to me they slow me down, get in my way. But in reality my limitations are the passageways to wisdom—that is, if I'm willing to learn from them.

What limitation are you resisting today? Headaches? Backaches? Upset stomach? Fatigue? Cramps in your calves? Don't bother resisting. It won't work. Instead, embrace your demon and listen to the wisdom being whispered in your ear. The area causing trouble in your life can be transformed into one of your greatest sources of insight.

Get a Hug

Our chests and abdomen serve us as sources of protection and power,
and as centers for nourishment and love. Watch a mother
nurse her baby, or visualize the way a child
rests its head securely on its father's chest.
—CARL KOCH AND JOYCE HEIL, *Created in God's Image* (1991)

When we love someone, our natural instinct is to hold them close against us. Somehow being close, body to body, allows for the transfer of nurturance and a sense of safety that no other physical gesture seems to provide.

In fact, researchers have found that the healthiest children are those who as infants were held up against their parents' bodies, chest to chest. Those children who were held off to the side of their parents' bodies or who were deprived of touch altogether became what researchers called "touch avoidant." By the age of six, these children would refuse nurturing touch. Those children who had been touched body to body however, welcomed safe touch.

Do you need to be held today? Find a person you trust and ask for a hug today.

Make a Change

*In addition to coronary and artery disease, many other kinds and
symptoms of stress damage can be traced back to the excessive
flow of adrenaline: headaches (tension and migraine),
gastric problems, ulcers, and high blood pressure.*
—ARCHIBALD HART, *The Hidden Link Between
Adrenaline and Stress* (1991)

Many of my clients are high-functioning and effective in caring for others. But when it comes to self-care, they draw a blank. One of my clients is a capable, professional woman (a morning person, usually rising at five A.M.) whose sister (a night person who sleeps until noon) used to call late at night to talk about her problems. Frustrated with her sister's intrusion and losing sleep, my client also developed stomach problems and caught the flu regularly. Her body was sending her strong signals. She turned her stress into a challenge by setting a series of reasonable goals for herself:

Week 1: Get an answering machine.

Week 2: Call my sister and tell her I'll talk for a half-hour, not during the workday, and not after ten at night.

Week 3: Use answering machine to screen calls and return calls when it's good for me.

In three weeks, she felt freed from prison! Yes, her sister got upset and tried to make her feel guilty. But my client held the line on these limits. Soon, her sister's phone calls decreased to a reasonable pace.

What is stressing you out today? Turn one stressor into a challenge by setting small, reasonable goals. You'll enjoy life so much more, and your body will be strengthened.

Let Someone Love You

It is hard for individuals in our culture to realize that true
independence is rooted in and only grows out of primary dependence.
—HARRY GUNTRIP, *Schizoid Phenomena, Object Relations and the Self*

With tears in her eyes, Lynda told the women in the support group, "I've gone as far with you all as I dare. I'm afraid to need you. What if I really start to trust you all, only to have you leave me like everyone else has?"

Lynda voiced what every other woman in the group felt. They were all afraid to believe that the others really cared. Many of us are afraid to trust because we did not have legitimate dependency needs met when we were children. Growing older doesn't make these needs go away. Rather, we move into adulthood, overburdened by the demands of unmet childhood dependency needs, with no understanding of how to satisfy those needs.

Our culture compounds the problem by defining independence as not needing anything from anybody. In order not to appear needy, we avoid depending on others for help.

Rather than view the healthy adult as a woman who is isolated and cut off from mutually satisfying relationships, we must acknowledge our dependence upon other people for our humanness and for the quality of our lives. Only with other human beings can we love and be loved, learn to have our needs met and help to satisfy the needs of others. What satisfaction does life offer without these experiences?

Take a risk and let another woman be there for you. Think of someone who has offered to help you. Call or write her a note and thank her for allowing you to rely on her care and wisdom. This woman has given you a great gift.

Ask Helpful Questions

I don't have all the answers—
I don't even have all of the questions yet.
—NANCY ZIEGENMEYER

I chuckle when I think about how sure I was of having it all together when I was a teenager. There were no questions I couldn't answer, if not to anyone else's satisfaction, at least to mine. But as I experienced more of life, my list of puzzling questions grew in number and the list of satisfying answers shrunk to an alarmingly tiny number. I've learned however, that if you ask a helpful question, you'll almost always come up with a helpful answer.

Our brains are designed to answer whatever questions we ask of it. If we ask, "Why can't I lose weight?" our minds will come up with a host of reasons explaining *why* we *can't* lose weight—this is not complicated. We'll hear our minds answer, "You're lazy," "You're a failure," or "No diets will ever work for you." What we'll never hear are any helpful ideas about how we could lose weight.

If you want to make changes in your life, ask a helpful question. Ask yourself, "How can I lose weight?" or "How can I stay faithful to my exercise program?" or "How can I cut down on the fat in my diet?" Then you'll get the answers you need.

Reveal Your Feelings

Truth is the only safe ground to stand upon.
—ELIZABETH CADY STANTON, *The Woman's Bible* (1895)

Ever have someone ask you how you're doing and you say, "Oh, fine," when you are anything in the world but fine?

We can lie with our words but not with our bodies. I can say I'm feeling great, but the bags under my eyes, the twitching of my left foot, and my shallow breath will let the world know I'm exhausted. I'll bet you've done the same thing. You can pretend you're not angry, but your flushed face, raised shoulders, and clenched fists will tell a different story. Or if you're trying to hide your depression, your slow walk and sad frown when you think no one else is looking will give you away. Your body will express what you cannot or will not express.

Sometimes I get so good at pretending I'm fine for the benefit of appearances, I fool myself. At times, I don't have a clue about what I'm feeling. If this happens to you, just take a look at your body and you'll find the truth. Your body will reveal what is really going on inside your heart and mind.

Take out your body journal and draw an outline of your body. Color in red all the places in which you feel pain right now. With a blue pencil, color in the areas that feel tight and tense right now. Last, color in the areas with green that feel relaxed and at ease. Observe what this picture tells you about yourself. Is your drawing covered with red and blue, with little patches of green? You may be in need of nurturance and relaxation. Or do you see a predominance of green on your picture? If so, celebrate how well you are taking care of your body and living in the truth.

Live Sensuously

We live on the leash of our senses.
—DIANE ACKERMAN, *A Natural History of the Senses* (1990)

Write in the numbers indicating how often, if ever, the statements are true. Modify those statements that don't apply to you. 1—Never, 2—Sometimes, 3—Always.

___I consider myself a sensuous woman.

___I use sensuous experiences to soothe, nurture, and inspire myself.

___I cope effectively if someone criticizes my sensuous activities.

___I attract sensuous people who share my self-nurturing interests.

___I believe that sensuality is a necessary component of life.

___I regularly enjoy music that soothes and/or energizes me.

___I regularly enjoy silence and solitude.

___I regularly enjoy natural fragrances like flowers and oils.

___I regularly enjoy visual experiences like photography, taking in the view, or watching films.

___I breathe through my nose, deeply and regularly.

___I am aware of what tastes good to me.

___I eat slowly, enjoying the taste of every bite.

___I regularly enjoy touch sensations like walking barefoot or wearing soft clothing.

___I include sensuous experiences in my spiritual life.

___I regularly receive professional massage as a sensuous pleasure.

Scoring Evaluation

37-45   Congratulations! You enjoy a life of sensuous joy.

26-36   Watch out. You aren't enjoying the pleasures available.

0-25   Body alert! Your senses are being neglected. Pay attention.

Imagine Not Knowing Your Dress Size

*There were no standardized sizes for women's clothing until the late
nineteenth century. Imagine never being asked your size.*
—JANE R. HIRSCHMANN AND CAROL H. MUNTER, *When Women Stop
Hating Their Bodies* (1995)

I saw another ad for a dieting program in which the woman,
slender and smiling, claimed to have gone from a size sixteen to
a size nine. I suspect every woman who sees such an ad envisions
what those two numbers mean. We've been tutored from adolescence
to look at a rack of clothing and know, almost instantly, the size
hanging there.

Not only can we envision the size of clothes, we also see the
woman who fits that size. We can estimate the shape of her hips,
the width of her waist, the span of her breasts.

Recognizing sizes would be of no consequence if value weren't
placed on those numbers. The woman in the ad didn't have to say,
"I was a size sixteen and that's bad. Now I'm a size nine and that's
good." The numbers are a judgment—small is better.

Only a few generations of women have been valued (or devalued)
according to their dress size. My great-grandmothers were probably
the first generation of women to suffer under this scrutiny.
Previously, women made their own dresses without a standardized
measurement. Focus was on dressing appropriately, not on squeezing
into a particular size.

Imagine being a woman who lived prior to the late 1800s, free
of TV ads telling you to be small, free of magazine images of
airbrushed bodies, free of beach films with adolescent girls. Imagine
enjoying the shape of your body simply because it is. Let yourself
be beautiful today, no matter your size.

Celebrate Your Belly Button

*Your mother loves you the deuce while you are coming. Wrapped up
there under her heart is perhaps the coziest time in existence.
Then she and you are one, companions.*
—EMILY CARR (1871-1945)

As a massage therapist, I see more belly buttons than your average woman might see. Some women refer to their belly buttons with affection. Others, who feel self-conscious about their stomachs in general, often have disparaging thoughts about its unique shape.

Belly buttons are a reminder that you were once fundamentally connected to your mother's body. Not only were you encased in her womb, your nourishment came through the cord of life that stretched between your tiny, growing body and hers. While you no longer depend upon another woman's body for survival, you will always be dependent upon the nourishment of other women to feed your feminine soul.

Celebrate your belly button. Celebrate your mother. Celebrate being a woman with the capacity to conceive and contain new life within your body. Poke your body buddy in the belly button and say, "Hey, ain't it grand to be a woman?"

Let Off Steam

Anger as soon as fed is dead
Tis starving makes it fat.
—EMILY DICKINSON, *Poems, Second Series* (1891)

Just about had it with everyone? Tired of all the demands? Ready to bite the head off the next person who crosses your path?

Before you let someone have it, sit in your car and yell. No one will hear you. No one will care. You can say all the mean, hateful, spiteful, outrageous, insightful, self-righteous things you want to say. And you'll never have to apologize.

Don't strain your voice. Just use it for what God intended—to speak your truth. Loudly!

Ignore Criticism

No one can make you feel inferior without your consent.
—ELEANOR ROOSEVELT, *This Is My Story* (1937)

Ever feel like you are selfish when you pay attention to your body's needs?

I certainly have. You can criticize me all sorts of ways and I can easily shrug it off. Tell me I'm stupid, too loud, an awful cook or worse housekeeper and I'll either agree with you and not care, or think you don't know what you're talking about.

But tell me I'm selfish because I get massages, that I'm self-indulgent because I enjoy bubble baths, or that I'm self-absorbed because I take time to reflect on what my body might be saying and I become paralyzed with guilt. Fearing any sign of self-care will be viewed as self-indulgence, I'll focus my attention on others and neglect myself. Whenever I let someone shame me into neglecting myself or misusing my body, I am giving the wrong people power in my life. I am considering the opinions of those who are not worthy of my concern.

What do you do with guilt feelings that arise when you take care of yourself? Just follow the advice of my friend Paula, who said, "Whenever I feel guilty for taking care of myself, I know I'm doing a great job!" Like Paula, redefine what guilt feelings mean and know that the guiltier you feel, the better you're taking care of yourself. Eventually your guilt meter will realign itself to include proper body care. Grant yourself permission to love yourself. Listen to those who support health, and learn to ignore the rest.

JUNE

SHOPPING LIST

One dozen eggs
One gallon low-fat milk
Apple juice
One smile from a friend
Unbleached flour
Iodized salt
One loaf of sourdough bread
Two hearty laughs at life
One box of Kleenex
One quart of bleach
One day of child-like awe
Cheerios
Diet Coke
One pint of wisdom-for-the-day
Bananas
Broccoli
Tomatoes
One small dispenser of joy
One head of lettuce
Five pounds of potatoes
One song of gratitude

Be Happy, Be Healthy

The dying process begins the minute we are born,
but it accelerates during dinner parties.
—CAROL MATTHAU

Much of our personal power lies, not in the extravagant or extraordinary parts of our lives, but in the little choices we make every day. Doctors James F. Fries and Donald M. Vikery write in their book, *Take Care of Yourself,* "Your lifestyle is your most important guarantee of lifelong vigor, and you can postpone most serious chronic diseases by the right preventative health decisions."

While I do not have the power to protect myself from all disease or mishaps, the quality of my health is greatly affected by the regular choices I make regarding diet and stress management.

According to the U.S. Department of Agriculture and U.S. Department of Health and Human Services, here's a list of do's for healthy eating habits:

♦ Eat a low-fat diet.

♦ Eat 3-5 servings of vegetables a day.

♦ Eat 2-4 servings of fruit a day.

♦ Eat 6-10 servings of bread, cereal, rice, and pasta.

♦ Eat 2-3 servings of milk, yogurt, and cheese (easy on the fat).

♦ Eat 2-3 servings of protein (beans, nuts, meat, poultry, fish).

But wait a minute. What about the stress of meeting all the rules? Study after study has shown that stress is a critical factor in health and longevity. In one study, 1,200 male business executives who were considered at high risk of heart disease were divided into two groups. The first half was given regular checkups but allowed to continue their lifestyle as is, while the second group was placed on a special diet with limited calories, sugar, cholesterol, and alcohol.

In addition, these men were educated about health risks and given regular checkups. The findings shocked the researchers.

The men allowed to eat as they liked had a significantly higher survival rate than those who were eating "properly." In fact, there were twice as many deaths in the second group than in the first. Why did this happen? One cardiologist said, "These results don't mean that you can stuff yourself silly with impunity. But my own feeling is that if a patient exhausted by effort and distress has his life invaded by doctors and other do-gooders wanting to constrain his eating and other behaviors, the hassle factor and loss of autonomy could prove the last straw."

I love that phrase, "hassle factor." If every time you sit down to eat there's a little voice in your head causing you to fret about potential disease, your stress level will soar. Rather than associate nurturance and pleasure with a delicious meal, eating becomes a frightful experience if not a daily reminder of one's inevitable death.

So take another look at the list and add these: Do exercise moderation in what you eat. But enjoy what you eat. Do your best to meet the guidelines, but don't take this all so seriously that you stress yourself out and really do some damage to your health. Be happy. Be healthy.

Be Fully Yourself

*Since you are like no other being ever created since
the beginning of time, you are incomparable.*
—BRENDA UELAND (1892-1985)

Ever compare yourself to some other woman? I suspect we all
do. Sometimes when I see a beautiful woman on TV, I'll think,
"I wish my eyes were blue, too," or "Her body is much better than
mine."

Comparing our bodies with other women's bodies is a fruitless,
self-defeating activity. In doing so, we exhibit spiritual anemia and
lack of appreciation for who we are in God's eyes. No woman has
ever or will ever have your eyes, your voice, your touch, your walk.
Rather than trying to be like someone else, take up the spiritual
challenge of being fully yourself. Only you can do it. Only you will
succeed.

In your body journal, list three things about your body that make
you unique and irreplaceable. If you have trouble with this exercise,
call your body buddy and allow her to help you. Others often see
attributes in us to which we are blind. Allow these special qualities
more opportunity to blossom by giving yourself permission to take
pride in uniqueness.

Shrug Off Stress

People who know how to enjoy themselves, always find leisure
moments, while those who do nothing are forever in a hurry.
—MARIE-HENNA ORLANDO (1792) in LYDIA MARIA CHILD,
Memoirs of Madame de Stael and of Madame Roland (1847)

Find a leisurely moment to release the weight of the world from your shoulders. As we rush around, keeping pace with life's demands, our shoulders often rise higher and higher. Slow down long enough for a "shoulder shrug" perfect for turning a hurried, hectic day into a calm, effective day.

Sit with your back straight. Notice the tension in your shoulders. Breathe deeply once or twice. On the next inhale, draw your shoulders up as high as they can comfortably go. On the exhale, slowly draw your shoulders down. Repeat this several times until your shoulders feel relaxed.

Eat Something Different

*When all is said and done, monotony may after all
be the best condition for creation.*
—MARGARET SACKVILLE, Introduction, *The Works of Susan Ferrier* (1929)

When you get bored eating the same old things over and over, spice up your diet by turning a ritual meant for weddings into a taste creation. By the end of the day, eat four things that fit the age-old tradition. Munch on something *old*, like a pickle or dried fruit. Chomp into the freshness of something *new* such as a fresh strawberry, newly baked muffins, or a bright orange carrot stick. Something *borrowed*? Make sure you share a meal with a friend and then talk them out of some item on their plate. And for something *blue* . . . this one is a bit more challenging since fewer culinary delights are blue. But keep your eyes open for blue tortilla chips, blue cheese dressing, or a blue plum.

Change a monotonous day into creative play. Invoke the unexpected.

Celebrate Your Bowels

"How do you know you'll think of another idea?" one customer asks.
My experience tells me more will come. My trust in
a deeper source of ongoing creativity is renewed as
I finish each pot and put my mark on it.
—MARJORY ZOET BANKSON, *This is My Body:*
Creativity, Clay, and Change (1993)

Ever been constipated? A wonderful experience, don't you agree? Ugh.

If our bowels hang on to waste and useless matter, our appetites can be affected because out bodies can't cope with the food already in our system. The cycle of nourishment slows down.

Our digestive system can teach us a great deal about the creative process. If we hold on to past fears, harmful relationships, and negative beliefs about ourselves we lose contact with the natural rhythm of creation, death, and rebirth. Rather than cling to the past for fear that nothing or no one else will come our way, we can learn from our bodies to trust and act in anticipation, before we are sure of the outcome. Just as our bodies eliminate food in anticipation of eating again, so we can shed old ideas and connections to make way for healthier ones.

What area of your life is plugged up today? Do you hate your job? Are you angry at a friend? Are you withdrawn from your mate? Or tired of your life in general? Follow your body's guidance and "let go" of whatever is holding you back. Make room for new nourishment. It's time for a "creative" movement.

Assess Your Stress

Why is life speeded up so? Why are things so terribly, unbearably precious that you can't enjoy them but can only wait breathless in dread of their going?
—ANNE MORROW LINDBERGH, *Hour of God, Hour of Lead* (1973)

I looked down at my legs and said, "Wow, look at those bruises! How did they get there?" From time to time I discover dark bruises on various parts of my body without any memory of when or how I received such a blow. These bruises signal me that I am moving too quickly, motivated by a sense of urgency that is causing me physical distress. In my haste to get things done, to run around town doing errands, to dash through my office dodging furniture, I'm ignoring the fact that my body is hitting, knocking, thumping, and whacking up against some very hard objects.

Pay attention to your bruises. Notice where they occur on your body and if you're aware when your tissue is being damaged. Take out your body journal. Draw an outline of your body and draw in the places you've been bruised. Let this picture remind you that your body deserves much better treatment than to be battered by neglectful movement on your part.

Know Your Body

If you think you already know everything you need to know about your body, think again. Otherwise, you'll remain stagnant as a lover, never expanding the possible dimensions of your sexual self.
—CAROL C. WELL, *Right-Brain Sex* (1989)

Fulfilling lovemaking is an interaction between two people who feel safe enough to be fully present with each other. Before we can be present with another person, however, we must first be fully present with our own bodies. How can we feel free to explore someone else's body if we feel reluctant to explore our own?

Before I received massage and body work, I was unaware of my skin. Massage helped me experience my skin as an avenue of pleasure and comfort. I discovered that the more aware I was of my own skin, the more adept I became at nurturing others through touch. The more touch I receive, the better I am at communicating my love for others through touch.

In your body journal, describe how you can get to know yourself better through touch. Try caressing your skin with a lotion you've not tried before, check out a book from the library to learn more about pleasuring yourself, or massage yourself in front of the mirror and notice what feels especially good to you. By becoming more aware of how touch feels to your skin, you can give more pleasure to your partner.

Hide Away

Treat yourself to what you need and want.
—ALEXANDRA STODDARD, *Daring to Be Yourself* (1990)

Working hard? Finding it difficult to have any moments of relaxation? Taking care of your body is especially difficult when at work, when traveling, or when you are stuck indoors with minimal space in which to move. In situations like these, I've found that I'm vulnerable to getting agitated and irritated, resulting in tight neck and shoulder muscles.

Even in the most confining of situations, a restroom is usually available. Excuse yourself for a short spa getaway. In the privacy of the women's room, close your eyes and imagine yourself at a glamorous spa. Let the warm water run over your hands as you draw air deeply into your lungs. Soak your hands for at least one minute, even two if you can. Concentrate on how the water feels on your wrists, hands, and fingers. Let the water run on the palms of your hands and feel the warm sensations. Then turn your hands over and feel the water on the backs of your hands.

Once your hands are warmed, place them on the back of your neck. First, hold them in place so that the warmth can penetrate your neck muscles. Take a deep breath and let the tension go. Once your hands cool down a little, gently massage the base of your skull, along the sides of your neck and, switching hands, over each shoulder, and down each arm to your fingertips.

Once you've massaged both arms, take a final breath. You will emerge from your spa getaway renewed and refreshed.

Survey Your Health

. . . [T]he body is all you can get your hands on.
—IDA ROLF, in DON JOHNSON, *The Protean Body* (1977)

Write in the numbers indicating how often, if ever, the statements are true. Modify those statements that don't apply to you. 1—Never, 2—Sometimes, 3—Always.

___I have a complete physical exam including a Pap smear and mammogram as often as my doctor recommends.

___I have my teeth cleaned at least every six months.

___I have a complete eye exam at least every three years.

___My blood pressure and cholesterol count are in the healthy range.

___My weight is within the healthy range.

___I have regular bowel movements.

___I brush and floss my teeth daily.

___I eat at least 5 servings of fruits and vegetables each day.

___I eat a low-fat diet.

___Every so often, I treat myself to something extravagant with no concern about calories, fat content, or being good.

___I drink at least two liters of water a day.

___I drink three or less alcoholic drinks per week.

___I don't smoke.

___I breathe through my nose, deeply, regularly, and calmly.

___I receive regular massage to strengthen my immune system.

Scoring Evaluation

37-45   Congratulations! You are taking good care of your body.
26-36   Watch out. Your body needs more care.
0-25   Body alert! You may be developing major health problems.

Motivate Yourself

It is not the horse that draws the cart, but the oats.
—RUSSIAN PROVERB

J ust do it! Right. We all know that one, don't we? If being good to our bodies could be accomplished merely by an act of the will, we'd be there. Rather than try to make yourself into a workhorse forced to perform according to your dictates, focus your creativity today on giving yourself "oats."

What's the hardest, least pleasurable thing you know you should do for your body? For me, it's eating broccoli. I know broccoli is good for me. Every time I turn around, some scientist is finding out something else beneficial about this green veggie. It's a source of vitamin C, vitamin B2, vitamin K, chlorophyll, iron, calcium, manganese, folic acid, and pantothenic acid, to name just a few. To get myself to eat this healthy vegetable, I reward myself with something special, like a fat-free frozen yogurt.

Identify your "broccoli." What is one thing you don't like doing that you know you should? Maybe it's exercising, taking naps, drinking more water, or taking your vitamins. Rather than heap mounds of guilt on yourself, find a reward that will properly and happily motivate you to move in a positive direction. Trade a less-attractive activity for one you love. Motivate yourself with a grand, sensuous reward!

Include All of Your Senses

Each day is a tapestry, threads of broccoli, promotion, couches,
children, politics, shopping, building, planting, thinking
interweave in intimate connection with
insistent cycles of birth, existence, and death.
—DEENA METZGER, *Heresies I*

A life well-lived encompasses all of ourselves—all of our senses, all of our feelings, all of our thoughts and desires. If you are like me, you've developed some of these areas but not all. And, sadly, like me, your body may have been the most neglected.

It's time to bring your life back into balance. Assess which areas need attention. If you're a reader, then put down your books for a while and simply smell the roses. Let your senses guide you through your next insight. If you live by your emotions, take time to study your body, think new thoughts, or read a new book. If you've been spending lots of time at the gym, take a break and carve out some time to pray and meditate. If you've been spiritually focused, get your hands dirty and plant a seed or bake a pie or paint a picture. Give all of your life the attention it deserves.

Celebrate Breathing

Good breathing is of utmost value in maintaining good body tone.
—GENE TUNNEY

The day before my last birthday I noticed that my driver's license was to expire the next day. It was too late to make an appointment, so I spent two and a half hours waiting in line at the Department of Motor Vehicles. As dozens of us inched our way to the next window, few around me were happy, to say the least. Frowns and irritation were the norm, with babies crying and eyes looking dazed in boredom. I could feel my throat constrict in frustration and hear that voice in my head, "How could you be so stupid as to not notice the expiration date and get an appointment? Look at those other people walking up to the window and leaving in a few minutes!"

Conscious of my body's agitated state, I knew I was heading for a miserable afternoon. So I tried something different. I decided to breathe. I took a deep breath to the count of six, held my breath to the count of twelve, and then released my breath to the count of three. After several minutes, I was actually feeling content.

Now it wasn't so wonderful that I'd ever want to do that again. The next time I have to renew my license I'm going to make an appointment. But I learned a valuable lesson about being stuck in long lines. Breathe. It doesn't bother anyone else, and it lifts the spirits and soothes the body. What have you got to lose but a frown?

Declare Your Space

Our sources and uses of power set our boundaries, give form to our relationships, even determine how much we let ourselves liberate and express aspects of the self.
—MARILYN FERGUSON, *The Aquarian Conspiracy* (1980)

How would you like to get on a plane and hear the pilot over the loudspeaker say, "Well, I've never actually flown one of these things before. I thought I'd just learn as I go?" I, for one, would head for the door immediately.

To learn skills, especially complicated skills that may mean life or death, requires and deserves practice. Setting boundaries is a skill that may save your life, so invest the practice time required to build confidence and mastery in setting your boundaries.

Stand in front of the mirror, looking yourself straight in the eye. Stand with your feet far enough apart that you have a solid foundation. Bend your knees slightly so that you can move easily in any direction. Raise your arms, holding your hands up and in an open position. First say, in a strong voice, "No. Back off!" or "Stand back!" Forget the neighbors or anyone else who may be within earshot. Practice in a strong voice several times until you feel confident.

Repeat this process, yelling the command as loudly as you can. Draw energy from the center of your body, using all the power inside you to declare your boundaries. Practice several days in a row, and then at least once a month, so that your body learns to move instinctively to position and your voice knows exactly how to sound should you be faced with someone who wants to harm you.

Explore Your Body

As children, we are naturally curious about everything in our world.
Our bodies are no exception; our exploration takes in all body parts.
—CAROL C. WELL, *Right-Brain Sex* (1989)

Do you feel free to explore your own body?
I remember with an uncomfortable giggle the scene in the movie *Fried Green Tomatoes* when women in a workshop are handed mirrors and instructed to inspect their genitals. I giggle because I am horrified at the thought of being in such a group, while still wanting to know what really is going on "down there."

Some of us feel apprehensive because we've been told, in subtle ways, that women should not explore their own bodies. Let's take back our bodies and support each other in the process. Here are a few suggestions:

♦ Take off all your clothes and observe yourself in a mirror.

♦ Gently rub your entire body with a fragrant lotion or body oil, noticing how each part of your body feels.

♦ Caress your breasts.

♦ Try a vibrator to reach orgasm.

Whether you're just beginning or have taken large steps toward making peace with your body, there is always more to explore. You're invited to be curious and investigate.

Follow Your Sleep Rhythm

Early to bed, early to rise, makes a man healthy, wealthy, and wise.
—BENJAMIN FRANKLIN (1706-1790)

D o you cooperate with your body's natural sleep rhythm? Sometimes following your body's rhythm isn't easy. No matter what our bodies want, we're expected to pop out of bed early and run to work, alert and ready to produce. As the day progresses, we're supposed to wind down. And, if we follow Benjamin Franklin's advice, we're asleep early and ready to go the next day.

Believe me, that doesn't happen with me. I am a night person. Boy, am I! We night people wake up groggy no matter what time of day we arise, and we gain energy as the day progresses. Unlike morning people who start fast and tire as the day goes on, we start slow and gain momentum. There's nothing wrong or immoral with being a night person. We can be just as productive, creative, and fun as morning people. It's just that our society is organized in the opposite direction!

Is your day structured around your body's rhythm? If you're a morning person, do you schedule your projects early in the day and give yourself permission to retire when you're tired, even if others pressure you to stay up late? If you are a night person, do you ease into the day and plan your productive hours for late afternoon or evening? The more you know your natural rhythm and cooperate with it, the healthier, happier, and more productive you'll become. If Ben lived today, maybe he would say, "To bed when you're sleepy, when rested, arise. Follow your body. Your body is wise."

Hold onto Your Inner Awareness

All this emphasis on money and acquisition can increase our sense of
insecurity and lower our self-esteem unless we focus on
what our needs and desires dictate.
—ALEXANDRA STODDARD, *Daring To Be Yourself* (1990)

Turning forty did me a world of good. My life was nothing like I thought it would be when I was middle-aged. I had intended to be living the 1950s version of the American dream—baking cookies for my children while wearing a pink apron and looking forward to my successful, handsome husband arriving home promptly at five-thirty. Suffice to say, my life didn't look anything like that.

Rather than be depressing for me, however, turning forty was liberating. If I were to judge my life by the standard I'd received decades earlier, I was already a failure. So what else was there to lose? Consequently, I no longer felt obligated to "behave myself" or worry about what others thought about me. After missing my goal, I had the opportunity to set new goals for myself, goals that were guided by wisdom gleaned from forty years of living and a growing awareness of my body.

Set your course by letting your body tell you what is important. Base your sense of worth and joy of accomplishment on hearing and honoring your body's inner wisdom—skills that endure long after prestigious cars, designer clothes, or any other outward display. Hold onto your inner awareness, and you'll never lose your self-esteem.

Turn the Radio On

It's not true that I had nothing on. I had the radio on.
—MARILYN MONROE, in *Time magazine* (1952)

B ack in the Garden of Eden, Adam and Eve ran around naked and didn't think to feel ashamed or self-conscious. Today, give yourself permission to return to the garden and enjoy your pure nakedness.

Create some privacy for yourself and get naked! Take an admiring look at yourself in the mirror and pick your favorite body part. Tell that part of yourself how much you appreciate all the wonderful ways it contributes to your life.

Oh, and if you would like to follow Marilyn's example, turn the radio on.

Locate Attraction in Your Body

*Flirtation is merely an expression of considered desire coupled with
an admission of its impracticability.*
—MARYA MANNES, *But Will It Sell?* (1964)

L et's face it. What fun would it be to flirt if you couldn't include
your body? So much would be missing without the seductive
smile, the rapid heartbeat, the batting eyelashes, the lingering gaze,
the casual brush of your hand. All the senses are involved in the
delicious art of flirtation.

How does your body express attraction to a potential lover? You
may know you're flirting when you catch yourself shaking your
head so your hair will shimmer, when your mouth is dry and your
lips stick to your teeth, or your brain feels like mush and no words
come out right. Pay attention while you flirt today, and record the
ways your body expresses your attraction.

Celebrate Taste

Every sociability can be found assembled around the same table:
love, friendship, business, speculation, power, importunity,
patronage, ambition, intrigue . . .
—ANTHELME BRILLAT-SAVARIN (1755-1826)

Taste is one sense that tends to draw people together. None of our other senses are shared in quite the same manner. We can enjoy how things look or smell or feel whenever the opportunity arises. But we tend to enjoy eating together more than alone, preferring to enjoy our taste buds and each other simultaneously.

Generate an attitude of gratitude for the richness of sensual delight and relational intimacy you enjoy aided by your sense of taste. And at your next meal with friends or family, take time to discuss this wonderful aspect of your bodies and pay tribute to the sense of taste!

See the Signals

If you can keep your head when all about you are losing their's, it's just possible you haven't grasped the situation.
—JEAN KERR, *Please Don't Eat the Daisies* (1957)

As I drove down a familiar stretch of highway late one night, the taillights of the car in front of me brightened red. I looked ahead and saw the flashing lights of police cars and a firetruck. I realized instantly what these signals meant—an accident. To keep myself from plowing into the cars in front of me and becoming part of the accident myself, I heeded these signals and slowed down.

Our bodies signal us about danger continuously. In the same way we are signaled through flares and flashing lights on the road, our body warns us of danger through sweating palms, a racing heart, a dry mouth, an anxious stomach, a pain in the neck. If we read these signs accurately and respond by protecting ourselves, we avoid unnecessary damage. If, however, we ignore these signals, we suffer. It's not very complicated, but for some reason, it's often difficult to do.

Taking care of yourself doesn't always require something dramatic. It may be as simple as staying out of the way of an abusive person or not taking the blame at work for something you didn't do.

How does your body signal that danger is ahead? Write down the specific ways your body reacts to threatening experiences. Then promise yourself that the next time you are signaled, you will respond by taking care of yourself immediately.

Cradle Yourself

How soothing is affection! And how do those who, like me, know
little of this sweetener of life, turn, with awakened tenderness,
to him who administers the cordial!
—MARGUERITE BLESSINGTON, *The Victims of Society* (1837)

Remember nursery rhymes filled with images of cradles gently rocking the baby to sleep? Admittedly, sometimes these cradles were rocking in precarious positions, as in the old song "Rock-a-bye-Baby." Nevertheless, the idea of a cradle was comforting to me when I was a child, even though I never had one. Like most of you, I slept in a stationary bed called a crib. Where did all the cradles go, with their gentle, nurturing rocking?

Believe it or not, in the late 1800s a professor from New York instructed parents to do away with cradles because he felt that babies should receive no physical stimulation! Babies were to be picked up only upon feeding (which of course was scheduled by the clock, not when the baby was hungry). So American families discarded their cradles and placed their babies in cribs that did not move or stimulate the babies' bodies in any way.

Do you need some affection and cradling today? Wrap your arms around yourself and rock, giving yourself the feeling of love and nurturance you may not have received as a child.

Cooperate with Nature

*The essential principles of health are not understood by all people . . .
and, alas! not by all our physicians, who as a rule have been
educated to cure disease, not to prevent it.*
—Ellen Swallow, *The New England Kitchen Magazine* (1893)

As was the case a hundred years ago, the focus of our health-care system is curative rather than preventative. As anyone can tell you who has been diagnosed with a serious illness such as cancer, heart disease, arthritis, or stroke, effort put into prevention is effort well-spent.

While we cannot protect ourselves from any and all illnesses, we can decrease the likelihood of succumbing to disease by strengthening our immune systems. Here is a short list of ways we can help our immune systems ward off disease:

♦ Tell the truth about how you feel.

♦ Say "no" the next time you don't want to fulfill a request.

♦ Eat your meals at a leisurely, enjoyable pace.

♦ Get your heart pumping three times a week.

♦ Drink fresh water every day.

In your body journal, continue this list. Write five additional ways you can personally cooperate with your body and strengthen your immune system. Then put these five actions into practice today.

Ignore the Irrelevant

The art of being wise is the art of knowing what to overlook.
—WILLIAM JAMES (1842-1910)

Stop for a moment and simply listen. What are the sounds you hadn't noticed? The sounds of traffic outside, birds tweeting in the trees, a cat meowing next door, the TV noise in the next room, the tinkling of wind chimes on the front porch. Bits of information bombard our nervous systems every moment. If our bodies were not designed to screen out most of this stimulation, we'd be overloaded with sensory input and unable to function.

Follow your body's wisdom in decisions you make—by carefully screening out the opinions, attitudes, and demands that overwhelm you or drain you of life's joy.

Pay attention to:

♦ Those who genuinely desire the best for you.

♦ Activities that energize and inspire you.

♦ Present opportunities for intimacy and creativity.

Screen out:

♦ Those who try to control you.

♦ Activities that leave you frustrated and depleted.

♦ Anything that distracts you from enjoying yourself now.

Open your heart to the gentle and loving voices that urge you to live a balanced, embodied life. When you hear a shrill criticism, do what your body does. Screen it out. Ignore it. Move on.

Embrace Fear's Energy

*We cannot escape fear. We can only transform it into a companion
that accompanies us on all our exciting adventures.*
—SUSAN JEFFERS

Ever read a story about someone who never tried anything new, had no challenges to face, and never changed? Me neither, because no such story would ever be published.

What interests us are stories about people who have faced challenges, most of which seemed impossible to overcome. Inherent in confronting new, sometimes overwhelming, situations is the necessity to deal with fear.

If we let our bodies be gripped by fear, we'll be unable to cope effectively with the challenges we face. But if we embrace the physical energy, open to the potent adrenaline pumping through our veins, fear can be channeled into decisive, protective action.

Fear, well-managed, gives us the energy to run from a potential mugger, stand up to a co-worker trying to intimidate and control us, or confront a family member who disregards our needs. Fear's adrenaline gives us the ability to speak up when it might be easier to be compliant and to set boundaries that might otherwise seem too difficult to enforce.

Think about the ways you effectively transform fear into useful energy. Describe a situation in which you channeled fear's energy to make needed changes in your life. Take a moment to feel proud of yourself for cooperating with your body's intent to protect you from further harm.

Be Ordinary

I often think, my dear, that it is a great pity you are so imaginative, and still a greater pity that you are so fastidious. You would be happier if you were as dull and as matter-of-fact as I am.
—EMILY EDEN, *The Semi-Detached House* (c.1860)

In a culture that rewards over-achievement and special skills, setting a goal of being ordinary can seem the equivalent of being unacceptable, talentless, lazy, or unlovable. But take another look at an "ordinary" human being.

The average person has approximately 206 bones, each of which can withstand a stress of twenty-four thousand pounds per square inch. This complicated, yet movable structure is held together with muscles, the strongest of which have a force of two hundred pounds per square inch. Surrounding the muscles is eighteen and a half square feet of skin, housing three million sweat glands that act as personal temperature regulators. The ordinary circulatory system carries blood (carrying twenty-five trillion red blood cells) through-out the body via sixty thousand miles of arteries, veins, and capillaries. If the ordinary person receives a cut, the platelets in the blood will start creating blood clots within fifteen seconds. Fairly amazing, is it not?

Go ahead, be ordinary. Be average. Be amazing.

Celebrate Your Stomach

Someone has said that the greatest cause of ulcers is
mountain-climbing over molehills.
—MAXWELL MALTZ

I'm convinced that my stomach and my emotions are directly linked. In fact, as I pay more attention to my body, I'm learning how to tell what I'm feeling emotionally by how my stomach is reacting. Tightness means anxiety. Loss of appetite means grief. When I'm hungry, I know I'm happy and relaxed.

Gastric problems, especially stomach peptic ulcers, are often exacerbated by emotional distress. Acids burn sores into the lining of the stomach and small intestines. This condition can become very serious if the acid burns through the tissue, resulting in holes in the tissue. Your stomach will let you know when you're working too hard, grieving a loss, or feeling great.

Celebrate your hardworking stomach today by paying attention to its needs. Record the conversation with your stomach in your body journal. If your stomach isn't feeling good today, ask your stomach what emotions are connected. And if you're feeling fine, treat your tummy to something yummy.

Claim Yourself

*Last evening we spoke of the propriety of women being called by the
names which are used to designate their sex. . . . The custom of
calling Mrs. John This or Mrs. Tom That, and colored men Sambo
and Zip Coon, is founded on the principle that white men are lords
of all. I cannot acknowledge this principle as just; therefore,
I cannot bear the name of another.*
—ELIZABETH CADY STANTON, letter to Rebecca R. Eyster (May 1, 1947)

When I tell people what I do for a living, I often get a few
raised eyebrows that say, "What do you mean you're a body
worker helping women come home to their bodies?" Suspicion often
fills the air.

There is something unusual, perhaps even frightening, about
women helping women unite with their bodies. Somehow our
bodies are supposed to belong to someone else—to our partners,
our parents, our country, our God. But claiming and naming our
bodies as our own, as our wise spiritual guides, is often met with
concern if not outright disapproval.

Resist the pressure to give your personal power to anyone else.
Claim your body as your own. Write a declaration in your body
journal that from this day forward, you are reclaiming responsibility
for your body with the intent of protecting yourself from the negative
opinions or physical intrusion of others. Share your declaration
with your body buddy to honor your decision to let all who approach
know that you are a united living force.

Make Your Move

Love is like playing checkers. You have to know which man to move.
—JACKIE "MOMS" MABLEY

Men are notorious for rating women by the shape or size of their bodies. So how about turning the tables by rating the men in your life—not by the shape or size of their bodies—but by how accepting they are of your body? A man worthy of your love and trust is a man who respects and honors your body.

Don't put up with negative comments about your thighs or weight or shoe size. Let him know that you love your body and you expect the same from him. If he is unable to love you, all of you, then it's very likely his negativity will push a wedge between you and your body.

Make room in your life for men who help you make peace with your body. And show the door to any man who is critical or unaccepting. Make your move.

Increase Your Pain Vocabulary

Even pain
Pricks to livelier living.
—AMY LOWELL, "Happiness," *Sword Blades and Poppy Seeds* (1914)

Ever have a small child come up to you and say, "My stomach hurts?" This complaint could indicate anything from an upset stomach from too much ice cream to gas pain to appendicitis. Most of us do not have a well-developed vocabulary to describe the pain we feel in our bodies.

Pain is one of the ways our bodies speak to us. In order to learn from our pain and make the changes our body indicates for a healthier, more balanced life, it's important to be conversant in the many ways our bodies feel pain.

Next time you say, "Ow, that hurts," take the time to describe the pain on a deeper level, drawing from this listing as a guide:

◆ Throbbing   ◆ Numb   ◆ Cutting
◆ Sudden   ◆ Aching   ◆ Piercing
◆ Shooting   ◆ Dull   ◆ Red-hot
◆ Traveling   ◆ Gripping   ◆ Cramping
◆ Tender   ◆ Sore   ◆ Vibrating
◆ Pressing   ◆ Tingling   ◆ Tender

Rebel

Being alone and liking it is, for a woman, an act of treachery, an infidelity far more threatening than adultery.
—MOLLY HASKELL, Film Critic

Enjoying one's own company can be viewed with suspicion. "Why is she by herself? Can't she get along with anyone?" "What's wrong with her, is she depressed?" "She actually told me she wouldn't go because she wanted some time alone. How rude!"

Being at peace with oneself is almost as unheard of as being at peace with one's body. For me, they are linked. When I am worn out, the best way for me to recharge my batteries is to spend time alone—alone with my thoughts, my feelings, and my body. All parts of me contribute to becoming replenished as I give myself time to let my dreams guide me while I sleep, time to let my mind wander as I walk, time to let my soul listen as I sit in stillness.

Rebel against the pressure to be an over-busy women. Instead, turn on the answering machine for the next few minutes and listen to what your body has to say. Listen to your throbbing feet, the pain in your lower back, the tingling in your scalp. Pay attention to the relaxing muscles in your pelvis and the soothing sound of your breath. The more you listen to your body's voice, the more you'll come to love it, and the more you'll live there.

JULY

BODY WORK

My body is
a work horse.

Carrying memories
of yesterday's
pain
my mind refuses
to recall.

Shouldering
the weight
of today's burdens
my heart refuses
to acknowledge.

Yoked to the promise
of tomorrow's
inevitable death
no part of me
can comprehend.

My body
is a work horse
pulling a heavy load.

Resolve the Problem of Pleasure

Every person has an agenda of worried private questions:
Am I enjoying the right pleasures? Am I having as much fun
as I should or could? Have I misunderstood what life—
my life—entitles me to?
—LIONEL TIGER, *The Pursuit of Pleasure* (1992)

There was no doubt to anyone within hearing distance that the twins, Nicholas and Alexander, were unhappy. After their parents researched the cause of their wailing, one was lifted to Connie's breast to feast happily and the other was wiped clean and soon gurgling with contentment in his father's arms.

Infants can be much wiser than grownups. They are attracted to pleasurable experiences such as wearing dry diapers, savoring warm milk, and sleeping when they are tired. Sometimes with loud protest, infants resist pain of any sort. The principle of pain and pleasure is clear to these tiny ones. Seek pleasure. Avoid pain.

We live in a society perplexed by a "problem of pleasure." Some are fearful of pleasure, linking this experience with inappropriate sexual activity. Many of my clients have asked me what I would do if they had sexual feelings during a massage. I tell them that all of their feelings are welcome in our sessions. Feeling pleasure, even if it has an erotic component, is a positive and safe experience. Experiencing an emotion does not dictate any specific action, however. Just as I would not allow someone to hit me if angry, I would not allow sexual activity to occur between us if sexual feelings arose.

A second response to the prospect of pleasure is confusion about who "should" or "should not" deserve a positive experience. Some people see pleasure as a reward for working hard or the suffering they have endured. They become uncomfortable at the prospect of enjoyment if a sufficient amount of pain has not been endured. This attitude, turned on its head, can result in fiery resentment if someone feels entitled to pleasure because they have experienced an excessive amount of hardship.

Some, I've discovered sadly enough, have lost their capacity to feel pleasure at all. Their bodies are painful to the slightest touch or completely numb, their hearts ache, and their minds are filled with worry. For these, pleasure has been eclipsed by the looming presence of pain in their lives.

Pleasure is not a luxury, but a requirement for survival. We are all entitled to pleasure, the same way an infant is entitled to nourishing milk, or the flower is entitled to sunlight. God gave us a body full of pleasure sensors by which to enjoy pleasure. We need not fear pleasure or earn it, but simply receive it.

Accept Balance

Peace comes from living a measured life. . . . My relationships are
not what I do when I have time left over from work. . . .
Reading is not something I do when life calms down.
Prayer is not something I do when I feel like it.
They are all channels of hope and growth for me.
They must all be given their due.
—JOAN D. CHITTISTER, OSB, *Wisdom Distilled from the Daily*

B alance is not a place at which we will arrive someday when things get easier. Balance is the path by which we make the journey. For example, I told a friend recently, "I'm so exhausted, but I want to do more on the manuscript."

"And you're the one telling people how to pay attention to their bodies?" she asked smiling.

"Yes, I'm the one. And leave me alone. I'm under deadline."

"Well, tell me, what is your body telling you now?"

"That I need rest, of course."

"Then rest," she said emphatically. "Rest."

Isn't there always something, if not several obligations, that seems to keep us from creating the balance we need?

I'll wait until I lose weight to go visit my family.

I'll wait until I can buy a juicer to start a healthier diet.

I'll wait. . . .

In your body journal, make a list of five activities you have neglected lately, activities that would restore balance to your life. Here are some ideas: straighten up a closet, eat your vegetables, get a manicure, schedule an afternoon to do nothing, or go window shopping. Join me in balancing and, if you'll excuse me, I'm going to take a short nap.

Celebrate Yourself

Nurturing is celebration, taking the time
to applaud being alive, being you.
—JENNIFER LOUDEN, *The Woman's Comfort Book* (1992)

How can you stand to touch me?
That's a question I often hear from my body work clients. Some women expect me to recoil at the sight of their bodies. We often believe our physical selves deserve ridicule or abandonment.

I know what it is like to feel embarrassed about my body. In fact, to protect myself from being judged because of my body, I simply pretended I had none at all. I lived in my head where I thought it was safe. I was wrong. After a total emotional and physical collapse from exhaustion, I wound up on a body worker's table hoping she could help me and that she wouldn't be repulsed by the cottage cheese on my upper thighs.

Instead of turning away from me, she treated my body with a respect I didn't have yet for myself. Her eyes saw the wonder and wisdom of my body, her hands heard the cries of my emotional and physical pain, her touch honored me. She started me on a journey toward respecting my body, and, in turn, I now share that respect with others.

I'm glad you are making your body a part of your daily experience. Make a commitment to yourself to celebrate your body in many ways. Celebrate your feet by dancing on your toes, your tongue by catching summer raindrops, and your skin by letting someone hug you. Marvel at yourself, acknowledge yourself. Ask your body buddy to give your body a standing ovation.

Vote for Your Body

The authority of any governing institution
must stop at its citizens' skin.
—GLORIA STEINEM, "Night Thoughts of a Media-Watcher,"
Ms. magazine (November 1981)

In 1777, Abigail Adams, a woman of prophetic insight, wrote a letter to her husband and co-author of the Declaration of Independence, John Adams, saying, "I desire you to remember the ladies and be more generous and favorable to them than your ancestors. Do not put such unlimited power into the hands of the husbands."

Unfortunately, her husband was not influenced by Abigail's admonishment. In her day, women could not vote. Most were financially dependent upon husbands or fathers. Wives were less partners and more possessions of their male family members, and fathers rather than mothers had legal authority over their children. A lot has changed since then.

We can vote, earn our own income, raise our own children, and exercise personal power our great-great-great grandmothers only dreamed about. As women who are in relationship with our bodies, we have a unique and necessary perspective on our nation's needs. As you decide how to vote in future elections, bring your body's needs and wisdom into the discussion. Which legislation protects the earth upon which our feet stand? Defends our bodies from violent rape and assault? Provides us with female-friendly health care? Our bodies require clean air to breathe, safe homes in which to rest, and fresh foods to eat. On this Fourth of July, ponder how your body can better inform your political decisions. In the next election, vote wisely. Vote for your body.

Remember What You'd Rather Forget

You need to claim the events of your life to make yourself yours.
—ANNE WILSON SCHAEF, *Meditations for Women*
Who Do Too Much (1990)

My client told me during a session, "I want to forget that ever happened! If I could just get that accident out of my mind, I know I'd feel better."

It's natural to want to avoid pain, especially memories of events or relationships that hurt us emotionally and physically. But the path of resolution does not take us through the Land of Forgetting. Only when we acknowledge and own our experiences, whether we chose them or they were thrust upon us, can we find peace of mind and body.

Describe in your body journal an event that you'd rather forget. Write down the experience in detail and then list the ways this event put you at odds with your body. Accept the fact that this event happened and that you suffered because of it. Nothing more is needed than accepting the experience as yours. Claiming your life, the painful and the pleasurable, will bring you home to your body, back where you belong.

Pamper Your Period

The fact that the majority of women in our culture suffer from menstrual camps is a very clear indication that we have something wrong with our relationship to our bodies.
—CHRISTIANE NORTHRUP, M.D., *Women's Bodies, Women's Wisdom* (1994)

Ugh . . . the cramps, the bloating, you know what I'm talking about. Most of us women, at one time or another, have had cramps at the beginning of our periods. If the pain is severe enough, we can wind up in bed a day or two each month.

A number of remedies have been touted over the years. Dr. Christiane Northrup claims that cramps are caused by many factors, so decreasing the intensity or duration of the pain requires a multi-faceted approach of diet, exercise, and decreasing stress levels. On a personal note, she acknowledges in her book, "When I become too busy or stressed out, I'll have a few hours of cramps on the first day of my period. They slow me right down and are a good reminder that I need to make some adjustments and to tune in to the wisdom of my body."

My personal favorite response to cramps is slowing down and decreasing stress by getting a massage. I let someone rub, smooth, knead, and pummel my aching, irritable body. Often menstrual pain is intensified by fluid retention and muscle tension, both of which are lessened through massage. Plus, getting a massage makes me feel pampered, which soothes my ruffled nerves, allowing me to emotionally relax and thereby physically release the clenching in my pelvic area. Welcome your cramps as a signal for change, time to slow down and receive some pampering.

Trust Your Body

Trust in yourself. Your perceptions are often far more accurate than you are willing to believe.
—CLAUDIA BLACK, Psychologist

When my life fell apart in 1985 due to colossal burnout, I didn't know what to believe or whom I could trust anymore. My faith in God was seriously damaged, as I had mistakenly believed that if I were doing good things for others, God would bless me and make my life work. When that didn't happen, I questioned my beliefs about God.

At first I thought I was abandoning God by exploring new ideas such as body work. But as my journey continued, I realized that God was leading me to a place of spiritual wisdom through healing the relationship with my body.

Now, over a decade later, I have a solid sense of trust in my body, not in place of God but as a conduit through which I believe God communicates to me. I can trust my body because God created my body and because my body reflects trustworthy, life-affirming love.

Whom do you trust? God? Yourself? Your body? Take some time today to reflect on your spiritual connection between yourself and God.

Be a Kid

The great thing about getting older
is that you don't lose all the other ages you've been.
—MADELEINE L'ENGLE, in *The New York Times* (1985)

Ever get tired of acting like a grown-up?
I do. And so do some of my friends. A while back, three of my women friends and I headed to the beach for a day of play. Getting on our hands and knees, we dug in the sand, molding high castle towers surrounded by deep moats certain to ward off any invader.

I never would have done this type of thing by myself, but surrounded by three other women (all of whom were therapists, by the way) somehow made it okay to experience my body the way I did when I was a little girl.

Gather your woman-tribe and do something fun and playful the way you did years ago. Finger paint, make mud pies, mold clay figures, play hide-and-seek. Remember your body from the past, and bring that joy into the present.

Locate Jealousy in Your Body

Jealousy, he thought, was as physical as fear;
the same dryness of the mouth, the thudding heart,
the restlessness which destroyed appetite and peace.
—P. D. JAMES, *Death of an Expert Witness* (1977)

I remember the last time I was fiercely jealous, several years back when I found out the man I was dating was also seeing a mutual friend. While he had every right to date other women (our relationship was not monogamous at that point), jealousy crackled through my body like a lightning bolt. My eyes narrowed as I gasped for breath. I felt torn from my moorings while simultaneously thrown to the earth.

How does your body carry jealousy? Are those hard knots in your forearms an unexpressed desire to wring someone's neck? Is that gurgling in your intestines the acid-filled thoughts about a rival? Are you clenching your teeth together rather than screaming your fears?

Take careful note of jealousy. Storing such an intense emotion in your body over a period of time can not only undermine your relationships but also threaten your health. Take out intense feelings on a pillow. Then use the jealous energy you find in your body to set safer boundaries for yourself and attract the secure love you genuinely deserve.

Celebrate Breathing

I am a restlessness inside a stillness inside a restlessness.
—DODIE SMITH, *I Capture the Castle* (1948)

How can your breath help you today?

Due to a misunderstanding, I recently had an unpleasant encounter with an acquaintance who yelled at me and then slammed a door in my face. Afterwards, I sank into a chair with heart pounding from anger.

I know myself, and I've learned it's much better for me to calm down before I speak angrily. I'm too eloquent when I'm angry, and then there are lots of apologies to make. So, realizing I was in a flooded state, I used my breath to soothe myself. Closing my eyes, I took several breaths. The first few were rapid and rather shallow because I was agitated. But as I continued, my breaths slowed down and became deeper. Once my breath was regulated, my anger was less intense. I was then able to devise a letter that clearly but kindly explained my position about the problem.

You can take charge of an emotionally-charged situation by inviting your body to assist in calming yourself down. Celebrate your breath today by watching for signs of being agitated or flooded. Regulate your breath to return to an alert state. In this calmer state, you will have full access to your problem-solving skills, your emotions, and your relational capabilities.

Assess Your Stress

There is an appointed time for everything.
And there is a time for every event under heaven.
—ECCLESIASTES 3:1, *New American Standard Bible*

Finding it difficult to find a time for everything you need to do? Feeling rewarded for your efforts or frustrated by the obstacles? You can answer this question by assessing your stress.

Take out your body journal and draw an outline of your body. Color in the tight and tense places, the irritated spots you notice. Maybe you've developed a rash on your thighs. Are you having trouble getting over that nagging cough? Maybe you're suffering from a vaginal yeast infection. All these signs indicate a stress level that's wearing down your immune system. Pay attention.

Compare this month's entry with preceding months to see what patterns or changes you can find. Do you have a tendency to carry stress in the same areas of your body month after month? Are you exhibiting tension in new places, in new ways? Becoming more aware of the ways your body suffers from stress is a necessary step in releasing tension and welcoming healthy relaxation.

Identify with Women

The art of being a woman can never consist
of being a bad imitation of a man.
—OLGA KNOPF, *The Art of Being a Woman* (1932)

Until the last several years, men served as a reference point for my femininity. I believed that my womanhood was defined by how well I pleased the men in my life.

Then I observed the men's movement and listened as the men in my life said, "We men have to meet together in groups to discover who we are as men. We can't look to you women for our fundamental masculinity." I realized that if this were true for men, it was also true for me as a woman.

Looking back now, I remember women inviting me to groups, but I saw no need for such gatherings. Of course not, when what I thought I needed would come solely from men. But now I am learning how to build my self-image as a woman on my relationships with women, and I am relating to men on my terms, rather than needing their approval for my sense of self-esteem.

Reach out to another woman today, a woman you admire for the way she holds herself and expresses her femininity. Take some time to invest in a deeper relationship with her. You will become more fully connected to your female body as you do.

Empower Yourself

I do not wish [women] to have power over men; but over themselves.
—MARY WOLLSTONECRAFT, *A Vindication of the Rights of Women* (1792)

Write in the numbers indicating how often, if ever, the statements are true. Modify those statements that don't apply to you. 1—Never, 2—Sometimes, 3—Always.

___I feel in command of myself and comfortable with my body.

___I ask for what I need in an effective, respectful manner.

___I insist on feeling safe and powerful in all relationships.

___I don't invest in relationships in which I feel overpowered.

___I don't invest in relationships with adults who feel powerless.

___When I am in crisis, my friends help me regain personal power.

___I breathe deeply, empowering my body with each breath.

___My posture expresses my personal power.

___I rarely waste time trying to change things outside my control.

___I feel powerful and comfortable when I express myself sexually.

___I rarely procrastinate, able to accomplish goals I set for myself.

___I use my personal power to protect and nurture my body.

___I work with my body to retain my personal power.

___I enjoy my work, feeling creative and rewarded.

___I have an empowering support network.

Scoring Evaluation

37-45 Congratulations! You are embracing your personal power.

26-36 Watch out. You aren't using all your personal power.

0-25 Body alert! You may be putting yourself in harm's way.

Get Rid of "If Only"

Regret is an appalling waste of energy, you can't build on it;
it's good only for wallowing in.
—KATHERINE MANSFIELD (1888-1923)

If only . . .
What a horrible way to start a sentence. Starting a sentence with these two words indicates a sense of powerlessness and defeat and dooms the speaker to failure and regret.

If only I were taller, I'd be happy.

If only my legs were thinner, he'd love me.

If only my breasts were bigger, I'd be sexy.

If only my skin were clearer, I'd be beautiful.

If only I had a perfect body, I would like myself.

Is there an "if only" in your life, giving you a false reason to dislike your body? Let it go, and instead ask yourself, "How can I be happy with my body right now?"

If you do, some surprisingly wonderful answers will come your way, courtesy of your body and mind.

Indulge in a Yummy Snack

Food is an important part of a balanced diet.
—FRAN LEBOWITZ, *Metropolitan Life* (1978)

It's easy to become so obsessed with dieting that we take no pleasure in eating. We must keep sight of the fact that eating can and should be fun as well as nutritious. Today's exercise is to combine low-calorie eating with a little bit of fun. Here is a list of ten yummy snacks you can have today that are each under one hundred calories:

1. 1 Fudgesicle (91 calories)
2. 1/2 cup plain non-fat yogurt with 1/2 cup fresh strawberries (86 calories)
3. 1 cup fresh pineapple (77 calories)
4. 1 slice of raisin bread (70 calories)
5. 10 jelly beans (66 calories)
6. 2 graham cracker squares (60 calories)
7. 2 cups plain popcorn (50 calories) (This is my favorite.)
8. 3 gingersnaps (50 calories)
9. 1 cup fresh strawberries (45 calories)
10. 1/4 cantaloupe (40 calories)

Don't simply eat one of these delicious snacks, enjoy every mouthful!

Take Your Body with You Wherever You Go

The body is shaped, disciplined, honored, and in time, trusted.
—MARTHA GRAHAM, *Blood Memory* (1991)

Ever live as if you don't have a body? I know all about that. I lose touch with my body all too often and go wandering off on my own. I make decisions out of my head, according to what I "should" do or what I think others expect from me. Without my body's wisdom, I get "addicted" to working too much and depriving myself of kindness and love.

My body's fairly patient, at least for a while, and then there's a headache, a bout of nausea, a sleepless night, or an irritable conversation with a friend. My body "whistles" to get my attention, and I realize, "Oops, I did it again. I forgot my body."

Many of us do it, leave our bodies out of our lives as if that were a real option. Ponder the question, "How do I leave my body behind?" Write the answer in your body journal. Perhaps you get so busy that you eat lunch around 3 P.M. or miss lunch altogether. Or you may race from one meeting to another and ignore your body's need to go to the bathroom until your bladder is in painful spasms. Ever work around the clock to meet a deadline only to collapse in bed for three days to recuperate? Today, take your body along, trust your body, and see the difference embodiment makes.

Celebrate Your Nose

Smell is a potent wizard that transports us across thousands of miles and all the years we have lived.
—HELEN KELLER, in DIANE ACKERMAN,
A Natural History of the Senses (1990)

Imagine some of the delightful fragrances and aromas of your childhood. Oddly enough, I revel in the aroma of fresh, moist soil instantly because it takes me back to making mud pies in the summer sun by the side of the house. I can't keep a smile away each time I catch a whiff of that earthy smell.

A whiff of chlorinated pool water transports me back to lazy afternoons playing with friends in our family pool. One of my favorite pool pastimes was playing Marco Polo, a hide-and-seek game any number of children could play together. Wafting over the water, I remember catching the aroma of corn on the cob roasting on our barbeque as my mother prepared dinner for me and my friends.

Celebrate your nose today by writing in your body journal how your sense of smell has reminded you of delightful past experiences. Identify specific smells, fragrances, and aromas that contributed to the pleasure of the event.

Deal with Danger

Acknowledging and believing in your strength of survival is what determines your ability to abandon yourself to pleasure without fear of pain.
—CAROL C. WELL, *Right-Brain Sex* (1989)

We do not wait until we're born to enjoy pleasure or to take action to protect ourselves from harm. Using ultrasound, seven-month-old fetuses have been recorded reacting to sounds and lights directed toward their mothers' wombs. At first their little bodies jump, startled by the noise, and all sucking motions cease. Often, they turn their heads in the direction of the auditory or visual threat, pulling their bodies into self-protective stances. Eventually, after the buzzer has rung or the light has flashed several times, the babies do not respond, apparently having decided there is no danger, and they continue their self-soothing sucking activities.

Imagine all the sounds that may have occurred around your mother—dogs barking, other siblings crying, an angry adult yelling, a car door slamming, fireworks exploding, TVs blaring. Before you were born, a barrage of scary, startling sounds made their way into the floating lagoon of your mother's womb. Most likely, the way your body responds to fear now is the way your body responded before you were born—curling your toes, hunching your shoulders, clenching your jaw, pushing away. You could have actually been born with knots in your neck!

Effectively dealing with danger is a task we are faced with from conception through the rest of our lives. Thank your body today for being there for you, naturally leading you toward pleasure and warning you of danger long before you can consciously remember, back when you were floating in your private sea.

Share a Secret

You cannot do it alone. And why try? There is real magic in each
person you know, and that magic is multiplied by the people your
people know (and so on). All that magic is just waiting to be tapped,
to enliven your life and help you fulfill your dreams.
—JENNIFER LOUDEN, *The Woman's Comfort Book* (1992)

Pizza face. That's what I was called as a teenager by mean-
spirited kids ridiculing my acne-covered skin. Even though the
pimples are gone, I still see myself as having a horrible complexion.

None of us learned to dislike our bodies by ourselves. To separate
from oneself is a learned skill, brought on by trauma, criticism,
disappointment, and rejection. In the same way that we were
wounded by others, we now need others to help us heal.

How would you like to feel about your body? Write a description
in your body journal of the feelings and opinions you wish you had
about yourself. Share this information with your body buddy. Be
courageous enough to share the dream and ask her to help you
make it real. You may find that she has a much more positive
perspective on your body than you do. Allow her affirmation to
increase your opinion of your body. With her support, acceptance,
and love, you can come back to your body and mend the broken
ties between your consciousness and your physical self.

Eat Some Water

Water is the best of all things.
—PINDAR (circa 522-443 B.C.)

Tired of drinking glass after glass of water? With a little creativity, getting the water you need can be more fun.

Some days I just can't stand drinking water—boring, bland water. Yuck. Even though I know it's good for me, I can reach my tolerance level for water, and I thirst instead for sodas and coffee and other less healthful drinks.

So, who says you have to "drink" the water your system needs? Did you know that you could eat certain foods that are comprised primarily of water and get the water you need?

Try a carrot, which is made up of eighty-eight percent water.

Or a cantaloupe, with ninety-one percent water.

A big winner in the water department is iceberg lettuce, at ninety-five percent water.

Tired of drinking? Then crunch, munch, and chew all the water you need.

Live in the Present

The present is the point of power.
—KATE GREEN, *Night Angel* (1989)

How much time do you live in the present? Review what you thought about today . . . an argument you had yesterday? The groceries you would buy tonight? The vacation you had last summer? The promotion you want next year?

Take a deep breath and come back to the present. All you have is the present. The past and future are outside of your power, but the present is fully available to you. Exercise the power of the present by living embodied, fully, sensually right now.

Take Time Off

All intellectual improvement arises from leisure.
—SAMUEL JOHNSON

Whenever I work on a manuscript, I forget that I can't be creative without the cooperation of my body. Trying to meet a publishing deadline, I push myself to write as quickly as possible. But eventually I get a leg cramp or a backache or a low-grade fever and my body reminds me that I've gotten off-track again.

So I stop. Take a walk. Browse through a used bookstore. Eat an ice cream. Pet my cats. Stretch out my back muscles. Listen to music. Spend ten minutes on my stepping machine. Relax and let my mind wander wherever my body takes me. Then bam, the next thing I know I've got a new idea and I'm excitedly writing the next section.

When you are stuck on a project, feeling like you can't possibly take another step, take time off. This is especially important when you don't have any time to spare, because you need your creative energy all the more. Take a few minutes, come home to your body, and you'll find a surge of enthusiasm and ideas.

Locate Impatience in Your Body

I have been devoured all my life by an incurable and burning
impatience: and to this day find all oratory, biography, operas,
films, plays, books, and persons, too long.
—MARGOT ASQUITH, *More or Less About Myself* (1934)

Tap, tap, tap . . . sigh, sigh, sigh . . . wiggle and squirm. These are all physical expressions of impatience. People reveal their impatience even when they are thinking about something else through the shaking of a foot, chewing on a lip, or leaning forward as if held back by an unseen force.

Keeping your body still is difficult, if not impossible, when you're impatient. It's much more likely that your body will express this tension long before you are consciously aware of emotional irritability. I've discovered my toes tapping, my breath held, or my body swaying, which leads me to recognize, "Hey, I'm tired of waiting! Let's get on with it!"

How does your body express impatience? This emotion is often carried through tension and expressed through repetitious movement. Get out your body journal and identify your unique way of communicating impatience in your body journal. After you're aware of the way your body carries impatience, express this energetic emotion rather than hold it hostage. Don't just sit there wiggling and squirming in your seat, stand up! Rather than impatiently tapping your foot, put all that energy into getting things moving in your life. Don't waste your time sighing. Speak up and say what you really feel. Take a cue from the impatience in your body and make a move.

Celebrate Your Sexuality

*All of us, children and adults, are beautiful flowers. Our eyelids are
exactly like rose petals, especially when our eyes are closed. Our ears
are like morning glories listening to the sounds of birds. Our lips
form a beautiful flower every time we smile. And our two hands are
a lotus flower with five petals. The practice is to keep our "flowerness"
alive and present, not just for our own benefit
but for the happiness of everyone.*
—THICH NHAT HANH, *Touching Peace*

I chuckle to myself occasionally when I see how generously
most Americans display flowers or use flowered patterns in
clothing or home decorations. I chuckle because the flower is the
sex organ of a plant. In general, our society is conflicted about
sexuality, and even the most liberated would not wear a dress printed
with penises or adorn bathroom walls with vaginas. And yet, without
any hint of embarrassment, we grow, wear, and fill our homes with
flowers. What a wonderful way to affirm sexuality!

Celebrate your sexuality today by wearing a flower in your hair
or putting one on your desk. No one will have to know (unless you
tell them) that your flower represents all the beauty, softness, and
fragrance of your sexual self.

Cast a Shadow

Unnecessary dieting is because everything from television and fashion ads have made it seem wicked to cast a shadow. This wild, emaciated look appeals to women, though not to many men, who are seldom seen pinning up a Vogue illustration in a machine shop.
—PEG BRACKEN, *The I Hate to Cook Book* (1960)

The visual messages surround us—be thin, be small, be weak. Whatever you do, don't be a power with which society must reckon. To use Peg Bracken's imagery, don't let your body be substantive enough to cast a shadow.

Rather than allowing the whims of commercialism shape your views about the shape of your body, invite a standard of health and vitality to influence your thinking. Rather than losing weight in order to achieve a specific body weight, eat a nutritious, low-fat diet, and your body will naturally slough off unhealthy, unneeded pounds. Rather than over-stressing your muscles, taking steroids, and depleting your energy to attain an idealized body type, exercise moderately and regularly. Your body will take its own natural shape with muscles toned, skin tight, and energy maximized. Rather than lusting after the "thin look" in the misguided belief that you will be lusted after, let your natural curves attract a lover who loves you for who you are, not for what you're trying to be.

Let your body be a powerful force in your life, guiding you to eating and exercise habits that will give your shape a full, healthy form. A loved and empowered body will cast just the right-sized shadow. Your shadow will reflect a powerful you.

Survive Disapproval

When we decide to heal ourselves we come up against some powerful forces. The first and most powerful is that our parents usually don't like sex and the belief is that as we heal ourselves and start enjoying our sexuality, then they won't like us.
—MARGO WOODS, *Masturbation, Tantra and Self Love* (1981)

The beliefs of our ancestors influence us, sometimes positively, sometimes negatively. Most would agree that attitudes about sexuality have, in the past, been anything but helpful. We seem to have to choose between being the madonna, respected but not sexual, or the whore, sexual but not respected. It's a tough choice to make, so I say, let's not make it. Instead, let's make a different choice altogether, that of embracing responsible sexuality that is both respectable and passionate.

Taking this course of action will need the support of at least one person you trust and who shares your perspective, such as your body buddy, a therapist, a body worker, or members of a support group. We all need this kind of support to cope with the spoken and unspoken disapproval we'll receive from society at large (and perhaps some of our relatives and friends as well).

Some people will disapprove of you defining your sexuality on your own terms. But you can bear their disapproval with the support of those who share your journey. Explore your sexual nature, be responsible, and be respected by those whose opinion is of value to you.

Catnap

Rest has cured more people than all the medicine in the world.
—HAROLD J. REILLY

A good friend of mine told me that when she used to work in an office, she'd get sluggish in the middle of the afternoon. Rather than go for the coffee machine, filling her body with unwanted caffeine, she would take a catnap in the bathroom. She found a restroom where there was minimal traffic, locked herself into one of the stalls, and fell asleep for a few minutes using the toilet paper roll as a pillow! Rather ingenious, if you ask me.

If you are tired, you probably need some rest. Be creative like my friend and find a way to take a ten- or fifteen-minute nap, even if you are at work. Unlike guzzling coffee, taking a nap will work with your body's natural process for replenishment.

Sense God in the Ordinary

The great lesson from the mystics . . . is that the sacred is in the ordinary, that it is to be found in one's daily life, in one's neighbors, friends, and family, in one's backyard.
—ABRAHAM MASLOW, *Religions, Values and Peak-Experiences*

Take a stroll through your own backyard (or around your neighborhood if you have no yard) and notice. Simply notice. Use your sense of sight and see the colors, the shapes, the beauty. Use your sense of hearing to take in the laughter of children, the roar of cars passing by, and the sound of your own breathing. Feel the ground beneath your feet as you walk, holding you with a secure hand. Notice the taste of your mouth and how the air feels as you draw in a breath.

Here in awareness is a beginning point for growth, a connecting point with the sacred that cannot be found through the spectacular or extraordinary. You are in your body. God is near.

Be Enthusiastic

We act as though comfort and luxury were the chief requirements
of life, when all that we need to make us really happy
is something to be enthusiastic about.
—CHARLES KINGSLEY

Stud, my rambunctious, daredevil cat, referred to by my friend as the "Gomer Pyle of cats," throws himself (literally) into anything he decides to do. The other day a fly got into the living room, an intruder Stud committed himself to capturing. Without concern for lamps, windows, or knickknacks, he repeatedly leaped into the air intent on catching that fly. The fly headed for the window, so Stud streaked through the air, smacking his head on the glass, while his flailing legs somehow found footing on an open shutter. Hanging in what seemed like midair, Stud batted the fly into his mouth. Twirling, he landed on all fours on the soft carpet, completely satisfied with himself.

I still smile thinking of his enthusiasm, the competent way he uses his body, and his complete belief in himself. So he looks like a fool from time to time. Who cares? He certainly doesn't.

Without throwing yourself into windows, lamps or other unforgiving objects, follow Stud's example of enthusiasm today and risk looking a little bit childish, foolish, or naive. Throw yourself and your body into your day with joy. You may end up with a scrumptious fly! (How's that for a motivator?)

Learn from Your Mistakes

There is nothing wrong with making mistakes.
Just don't respond with encores.

—ANONYMOUS

Oh, no. . . . I've done it again! I abandoned my body, became too stressed, and wham! Another migraine.

So, what do I do now? Lie in bed and fume at myself? No, that will get me nowhere. What is important is to accept the fact that I've made a mistake and learn whatever lessons my body wants to teach me. Obviously I've something important to learn, or I wouldn't be forced out of my regular routine by the pain.

Have you messed up lately? Did you carry a box you knew was too heavy and pull your back out of alignment? Did the temptation to eat sugar get the best of you when your aunt showed up with a plate full of brownies? Did you get so busy last week you completely ignored your exercise routine? That's okay. We all make mistakes. Don't waste your time heaping blame upon yourself. Instead, take this opportunity to learn something from experience. Learn to ask for help when the load you are carrying is too heavy. Be honest with your aunt about your infatuation with sugar and ask her to show her affection in other ways. Set clearer limits on your time this week, placing a higher priority on your physical well-being. When we learn from our mistakes, we turn them into successes.

Celebrate Your Arms

Your thorns are the best part of you.
—MARIANNE MOORE, *Selected Poems* (1935)

When I was a teenager, I overheard another girl make fun of me by hooting and dragging her arms like a chimpanzee. My arms are about an inch longer than the norm, so it's impossible to find long-sleeved blouses that fit. I usually roll up the sleeves as a "fashion statement." To get jackets that fit, sometimes I have to buy an entire size larger. Otherwise my wrists hang below the sleeves, making me look like I've outgrown my clothes.

Some of my women clients feel self-conscious about their arms because they are hairy. Since the ideal woman's body has little or no body hair, we sometimes feel less feminine if hair adorns our arms. Others are embarrassed if their skin is freckled, wrinkled, or splotchy. A few of my clients have suffered serious car accidents in which their arms received deep cuts or burns. Years after the accident, these scars serve as a reminder of the trauma and a point of self-consciousness about the acceptability and beauty of their arms.

No matter how hairy or long or splotchy they may be, our arms are a vital part of who we are. With our arms, we hug our children, carry our groceries, embrace our mates, protect ourselves from assault, and give our hands a place to live.

Celebrate your arms today. Bring out your body journal and draw a picture of your arms. Talk to your arms, expressing both your positive and uncomfortable feelings. Thank your arms for all the wondrous parts of life you enjoy through them.

AUGUST

ARCHAEOLOGIST

Sahara sands
swept across
crags and crevasses:
flattened the terrain;
covered rage, shame,
longing, hope.
Left nothing but
smooth desert death.

It is time to excavate,
again.

Don't Scare Yourself

*Many a man who would not dream of putting too much pressure on
his automobile tires lays a constant overstrain
on his heart and arteries.*
—BRUCE BARTON

Since there are plenty of things to frighten us in this world
today—crime, disease, economic uncertainty, war—why make
matters worse by scaring ourselves? I am very skilled at getting myself
worked up over the smallest thing. There's no one more
accomplished at agitating me than I am.

When I'm at odds with my body, I forget to focus on activities
or experiences that soothe me. Instead, I tend to do the very things
that will agitate me even more, such as over-committing to work
deadlines, raging over time pressures, and canceling social outings
that would renew me. Getting involved in relationships with men
who are a bit dangerous and unpredictable is another way I agitate
myself. Telling myself that I'm going to go broke soon and end up
a bag lady is a favorite way of getting the adrenaline pumping.
These agitating thoughts scare me into forgetting my needs, and
they distract me from taking responsibility for living my life well.

What scary things do you tell yourself? Get out your body journal
and write these phrases down. You may want to discuss these with
your body buddy to gain perspective on how helpful or harmful
frightening self-talk is for you. Make a commitment to talk kindly
to yourself, assuring yourself with statements that are soothing and
life-enhancing.

Live in Integrity

I like to deliver more than I promise instead of the other way around.
Which is just one of my many trade secrets.
—DOROTHY UHNAK, *The Investigation* (1977)

I want to think of myself as an honest woman, someone who tells the truth and can be relied upon when I give my word. But sometimes I run into trouble in my relationships because I have promised more than I deliver. Even though I mean to follow through on my commitments, it's easy to underestimate how much time a particular project will take or overestimate how much time I have to give. My good intentions don't lessen the disappointment experienced by others when I let them down.

Living outside of integrity will damage any relationship we have—with our girlfriends, our spouse, our children, or our co-workers. Perhaps the relationship that is damaged with the most frequency is the one we have with our bodies. I have lost track of the times I've promised my body I will take more time to rest, the times I've started an exercise program and then let it drop after a few weeks, or the times I've meant to eat better but then those deep-fried appetizers appeared before my eyes. I meant to follow through on my promises to my body. I really did. But time and again my body has been disappointed in me.

If you have broken your word with your body, write a letter of apology to your body in your body journal. Read it out loud so that you and your body can hear. Ask your body how you can make amends for living outside of integrity. And before you make another promise to your body, be sure that you are able and willing to keep your word.

Give Yourself the Once-Over

*No tissue is more adaptable than the skin. From the firm velvetiness
of the infant to the dry and wrinkled parchment of old age,
it is undergoing constant changes
in its size, shape, qualities, and functions.*
—DEANE JUHAN, *Job's Body* (1987)

Every so often I take off all my clothes and give myself the once-over in the mirror. This may seem like an odd activity, but I am checking for changes in my skin. Being fair-skinned, I am more likely than some to develop various forms of skin cancer, and it is important to keep up to date on my skin condition.

I pay special attention to any moles I have, especially those regularly rubbed by clothing (like under my bra strap) or those that get a lot of sun (like the one I have on my neck that is always accessible to the light). A couple of times a mole has turned black or has reddened around the edges, and I've had these removed. Fortunately, they have been benign. But as with any form of cancer, early detection offers the best chance for a cure.

Get nude today! Give yourself the once-over as a way to affirm yourself and contribute to your health.

Be Beautiful

We all share beauty. It strikes us indiscriminately. . . . There is no
end to beauty for the person who is aware. Even the cracks between
the sidewalk contain geometric patterns of amazing beauty.
If we take pictures of them and blow up the photographs,
we realize we walk on beauty every day,
even when things seem ugly around us.
—MATTHEW FOX, *Creation Spirituality* (1991)

Beauty is a word usually reserved for a select few—the supermodels or movie stars—women most of us will never be. Used as an advertising device, beauty is presented as a goal to be achieved through purchasing expensive creams, through applying just the right makeup, or through exercising on a particular piece of equipment. Why do we allow ourselves to be so powerfully influenced by those who sell us things through convincing us we are unacceptable and un-beautiful?

Beauty is not a thing to be bought by the masses or endowed on the few. Beauty is all around us. Beauty is in us. We are beauty. We only need to look at ourselves with new eyes, refusing to accept the superficial definitions given to us by the media. Open yourself to a new thought—that you are already beautiful. No need to struggle. No huffing and puffing. No applying or scrubbing. Simply be beautiful. Simply be.

Take a Risk

Take a risk a day—one small or bold stroke that will
make you feel great once you have done it.
—SUSAN JEFFERS

Stud, my white-whiskered black cat, stands at the door and cries in the late afternoon. By that time of day, he's torn up all the papers he could find in my office (or at least the important ones), he's taken his nap in the upstairs bathroom sink where it's nice and cool, and he and Sassy, my all-black female feline, have chased each other up the stairs, through the bedroom, into the office, back down the stairs and into the living room enough times to get on Sassy's nerves and have her hiss at him. So, by the late afternoon, he gets a bit bored and cries to be let into the yard where new adventures are waiting.

We've all got a little Stud inside of us, that part of us that longs for more adventures and new excitement. Not only do we have an emotional need for stimulation, our bodies need challenges as well. Researchers have found that baby animals that receive no stimulation or challenges are no better prepared to deal with life effectively than those who are overwhelmed with stressors. We need a certain level of stress coupled with a realistic chance of success in order for our bodies to develop fully. Adventures keep us healthy and happy.

So, listen to your body's desire for something new. Pay attention to that part of you that, like Stud, is sitting by the front door, crying for a little excitement. It's okay to let yourself take "safe" risks. Just keep an eye on the front door as you venture into the challenge of trees, squirrels, bugs, and neighborhood dogs. Pick your adventures wisely, just the way I do for little Stud.

Take Your Body on Vacation

*I will tell you what I have learned for myself. For me, a long five or
six mile walk helps. And one must go alone and every day.*
—BRENDA UELAND (1892-1985)

Do you include your body in your times of solitude and
renewal? I benefit so much more from my time alone if I
include activities that involve my body.

One of my favorite activities is walking through the Huntington
Gardens, a large estate in Pasadena full of luscious plants, flowers,
and various kinds of gardens. I feel my feet make contact with the
earth, I breathe the sweet aroma of the flowers into my lungs, I
listen to the birds and wind, and I let my eyes drink up the beauty.
This form of solitude not only invigorates me physically but also
renews my spirit, soothing any bruised emotions and stirring up
new creative energy.

Solitude is one of the many avenues of making peace with our
bodies. Next time you have a free moment, take your body on a
walk. You and your body will come back a bit more in sync and a
little less suspicious of each other.

Celebrate Your Senses

Too much of a good thing can be wonderful.
—MAE WEST (1892-1980)

Ever find yourself depriving yourself of something fun, nourishing, wacky, and wild just "because?" Dive into the deep end, roll around in the clover, drink until your thirst is quenched, and take in all the goodness life has to offer. Today, meditate on ways you can take in more of the exciting, enchanting, exhilarating experiences available to you!

What can I do today to make my
skin satisfied?
tongue whistle for joy?
ears perk up?
eyes grin?
nose wiggle with pleasure?

Assess Your Stress

Sometimes I wish I had suction cups to hold me down.
—PAM, in ANNE WILSON SCHAEF, *Meditations For Women
Who Do Too Much* (1990)

Sometimes I wish that some force bigger than myself would simply make me take better care of my body. Especially when I look back over choices I've made and realize that, once again, I've gotten off-track.

Get out your body journal and find a clean sheet of paper. Draw an outline of your body and then color in the areas of your body that are carrying stress. Your wrists may ache, your skin may itch, your thighs may cramp. Mark all the areas you notice.

Now compare this month's drawing with last month's. Are you carrying stress in similar places? Do you have any new locations? Are parts of your body more relaxed than last month? Keep your drawing so that you can see how stress affects your body on a long-term basis.

Take in Touch

We touch heaven when we lay our hands on a human body.
—NOVALIS, in THOMAS CARLYLE, *Miscellaneous Essays, Vol. II* (1772)

When my great-grandmother was born in the late 1800s, she had only a fifty percent chance of living past the age of two. Had she been placed in an orphanage, her chance of survival would have dived to a mere twenty-five percent. Why would so many babies die?

The medical community of that day promoted cleanliness to avoid contact with bacteria. The religious community preached strong discipline so that children would grow into moral citizens. Parenting experts strongly advised against touching children as they believed such doting would lead to emotional problems. So parents and orphanages provided these babies with clean surroundings, adequate food, plenty of discipline, and no touch. As a consequence, many infants died from a disease called marasmus, which means "wasting away." They died from lack of touch.

Those of us who lived into adulthood received enough touch to survive infancy. But we may not have received all the touch we need. Did you receive the touch you needed?

Look over family pictures to see how you were touched as a child. Are you being cuddled, or held limply by someone who seemed uncomfortable or disinterested? As you grew older, are you and your family members touching each other in a relaxed manner, or standing side by side like cardboard soldiers? Do the pictures reveal a family that embraced each other or one that kept each other at arm's length? Do you lean in or away from the person beside you? Discuss with your body buddy the nurturing touch you did or did not receive as a child, and how this affects you today.

Cooperate with Healing

Every living thing has a life force, energy or "soul" which is
impossible to get hold of or to see. . . . It is this life force which is
there even when our bodies are in poor health, giving us
the strength to try to regain normal health.
—SHIRLEY RICE, *Practical Aroma Therapy* (1994)

Not long ago I contracted a sinus infection that landed me in bed. Normally, these bouts last a week or more, sometimes keeping me in bed for three weeks. This time, however, I was up and around in three days because I changed my response to the illness.

Rather than pretend I wasn't sick, I quickly accepted the illness as fact. I called the people with whom I had appointments for the next few days and rescheduled, so I wasn't feeling pressured to meet normal work demands. And then I went to bed.

Released from stress, I listened to what my body had to say. I decided to make a significant change in my work situation, a stressor that I believe contributed to my decreased immune system. Within three days I was back at work, with a new vision I received by listening to my body, rather than complaining about my body through my recovery.

We all have a life force within us, whether we are sick or well, that endeavors to lead us to healing and understanding. I believe this force originates in God and is meant to guide us. While I'm not grateful for my illness, I am indebted to the wisdom I received while lying in bed listening to the voice of God.

Exhaust Yourself with Fun

To live exhilaratingly in and for the moment is deadly serious work,
fun of the most exhausting sort.
—BARBARA GRIZZUTI HARRISON, *Off Center* (1980)

So much in our society today pulls us toward an attitude of cynicism and despair. Resisting that tide takes a conscious decision and a great deal of effort. Being open to new possibilities, when those around you scoff at your naiveté, requires strength of character. Abandoning yourself to play when others are mired in depression takes courage. Trusting your body to lead you in a society that worships logical, linear thought can trigger ridicule.

Take out your body journal and describe something daring you've wanted to do but haven't yet mustered up the courage to begin. Maybe you've wanted to take ballet lessons but are afraid you'll be criticized for starting later in life. Perhaps you've imagined yourself in a drastically different hair style or color but have been reluctant to risk the reaction. Maybe you've wanted to attend massage school but those around you think massage is kinky, weird, or even immoral. Have you wanted to climb a mountain to the top? Take up skin diving? Take a class in vegetarian cooking?

Ask your body to help you deal with the criticism others may throw your way. For extra support, share your dream with your body buddy. Go beyond what most people achieve. Live positively, live in your body, exhaust yourself with fun.

Bathe in Iced Tea

The worst sin—perhaps the only sin—
passion can commit, is to be joyless.
—DOROTHY L. SAYERS, *Gaudy Night* (1935)

Prepare for a hot summer night by making a pot of chamomile tea and pouring it into an empty ice cube tray. Allow it to freeze. When the night air is smoldering, take the ice cube tray and draw a hot bath. Add a squirt of your favorite bubble bath, and let the foam fill the tub.

Sink into the hot water and bubbles, allowing your temperature to rise even more. Take an ice cube from the tray and rub it all over your body, above and below the water line. It won't take long before all the cubes will have melted, leaving your body tingling with delight. For more passion, invite your partner to join you. A joyful way to spend a hot summer's eve.

Locate Confidence in Your Body

I am filled with confidence, not that I shall succeed in worldly
things, but that even when things go badly for me
I shall still find life good and worth living.
—ETTY HILLESUM, *An Interrupted Life:*
The Diaries of Etty Hillesum 1941-1943 (1983)

Confidence gives us the courage to move into the unknown, certain we can handle whatever may come our way. An emotion easy to spot in a person's body, confidence shows itself in the tilt of our chins, the gleam in our eyes, the line of our posture and the power of our stride.

Get out your body journal and describe how confidence expresses itself through your body. Do you draw breath into your lungs with enthusiasm? Is your spine straight and tall? Is there a smile on your lips? Take a look in the mirror and see the confidence in your body, and you'll discover why others believe in you when you're sure of yourself.

Celebrate a Body Part

*It is because we sense love's power to transform that we are constantly
seeking to be in its midst, to partake of the blessings it can confer.*
—DAPHNE ROSE KINGMA, *True Love* (1991)

I once dated a man who told me he didn't think our relationship
could work because my ankles were fat. I tried to defend myself
against this cruel assault, but to tell the truth, I looked at my ankles
differently after that relationship ended. I didn't appreciate them
the way I had in the past.

I dated another man who told me that he loved my legs and felt
proud to be seen with me. His kindness, his love helped mend the
relationship I had with my ankles. I brought them out of hiding
and was once again able to thank them for the many wonderful
ways they contribute to my life.

The moral of these stories? Celebrate a part of your body that
has been criticized by someone else. Open yourself up to
compliments about this body part. Let love transform and mend
your relationship with your body. (And be careful about whom
you date.)

Banish Fear with Rituals

Working with plants, studying colorful gardening and bulb catalogs,
strolling through a fragrant arboretum: what a calming, refreshing,
life-affirming way to comfort yourself!
—JENNIFER LOUDEN, *The Woman's Comfort Book* (1992)

As I walked to my front door one evening, I found myself staring down a gun barrel, held by a ski-masked man who demanded my purse. I gave it to him. Fortunately, that's all he wanted. The police were responsive; my neighbors protective, my friends supportive, my parents alarmed. And I? I was cool, calm, and collected—and refused to leave my home for two weeks.

Eventually I emerged back into the world, at first only by daylight. Slowly, usually with someone accompanying me, I regained a sense of safety navigating at night.

To mark my physical survival and emotional healing, three dear women friends joined me in a ritual. We burned sage along the path I took when mugged to symbolically reclaim my space. To mark my release of fear and anger, we shared a cleansing drink (I'd intended to use chamomile tea but got talked into Diet Coke instead!). The ritual ended with each woman presenting me with a plant, bringing new life into my home.

The plants from this ritual offer me sensual reminders that I am loved and have survived a frightening experience. My eyes enjoy the mixture of greens and shapes, my nose enjoys the fragrance of the blooms, and my fingers delight in the feel of the soil.

We all undergo frightening experiences. Ask friends to help you regain a sense of personal power by sharing a ritual that includes plants. Plants nurture your senses, help you heal, and celebrate the healing.

Take Time for Simple Pleasures

Time for a little something.
—A. A. Milne (1882-1956)

Simple pleasures are often the most satisfying, especially if they are shared with someone you love. Invite a loved one to take a few moments to enjoy a simple pleasure incorporating one or more sensory channels. Here are a few ideas:

♦ Sun by the pool while sipping a delicious fruit drink and gazing into the eyes of your beloved.

♦ Hike up a mountain trail while chatting with your partner and admiring the view.

♦ Dance cheek-to-cheek to your favorite romantic music.

♦ Eat a mango together.

♦ Share a pot of fresh vegetable soup.

Share a simple pleasure through the wonders of your senses.

Ease Your Eyestrain

Our eyes need light to see. Healthy eyes depend, however, on open minds in order to see clearly. . . . Maybe a way of seeing all of life more fully is to start by marveling at our own eyesight.
—CARL KOCH AND JOYCE HEIL, *Created in God's Image* (1991)

I remember taking a computer class in college a long time ago when computers were huge and unfriendly to a right-brainer like myself. The professor of the class told us that in our lifetimes most homes would have computers. Ugh, I thought, I could never work on a computer. Never. And here I sit, some years later, pecking away on my PC, fulfilling the prophecy of my college days.

More and more people are using computers in their professional and personal lives. Consequently, more and more people are suffering eyestrain from staring at the computer screen hour after hour.

Take notice that your eyes are working very hard for you. Thank them by easing eyestrain: Reduce monitor glare by facing the monitor away from windows. Keep your paperwork nearby and at monitor level to reduce the amount of refocusing required. Blink your eyes regularly so that they will remain moist and cleansed. Give them a break by regularly looking away from the screen and paperwork.

Celebrate your eyes by caring for them with common sense and kindness.

Worry Once a Day

A request not to worry . . . is perhaps the least soothing message capable of human utterance.
—MIGNON C. EBERHART, *The House on the Roof* (1934)

Don't you hate it when people tell you not to worry? Just being told not to worry worries me. I mean, if there weren't anything to worry about, why would someone tell me not to? Try as I may, I suspect I'll always worry.

One way I've been able to put some boundaries on my worrying and limit the stress this useless activity creates for my body is to give myself a fifteen-minute worry break each day. For that period of time, I am free to worry, fret, fuss, and fume all I want. No guilt. No attempts to contain myself, just full-out, free-for-all worrying. What a blast!

And then, I stop. If a worried thought comes into my mind, I tell myself, "Wait until tomorrow, and you can worry about this then." Oddly enough, most of the time this promise to worry in the near future is all it takes to get my mind to release the troublesome thought. Of course, I have to make sure I keep promises I make to myself and indeed take fifteen minutes to worry the next day. Otherwise, I stop trusting myself and worry all the time.

So, if worrying has gotten the best of you (you'll know because if you listen your body will tell you), then set aside a specific amount of time each day and worry wildly. The rest of the day you'll be able to set your mind to problem-solving, getting things done, and enjoying your life.

Follow Creativity

*Art is a mystery. When I start a picture, I don't know no more what
I'm going to do than you do.*
—MINNIE JOENS EVENS

Some mornings I put on inspirational music and dance a prayer
to God. Without practice or preconceived ideas, my body moves
easily and freely around my living room expressing emotions that
transcend words. Creative movement frees me momentarily from
the stresses of the day. When I am finished with my prayer, I feel
refreshed and spiritually grounded.

Following the creative force within our bodies sets us off on a
journey most in our society don't share. Some do not believe the
body has wisdom, rather "it" is a mechanism to be controlled. Others
fear this approach because it is so mysterious and uncontrollable.
And, indeed, the body is uncontrollable.

Rather than try to control your body, allow your relationship
with your body to be led by the mystery of creativity. Treat your
body as an artistic expression, and allow yourself to discover yourself
as you go.

Live Your Dreams

Who's stopping you?
—ALEXANDRA STODDARD, *Daring To Be Yourself* (1990)

If you fully expressed who you are as an individual, would you be living the way you do now? Would you be in the same job? Would your schedule look the same? If the answer is "yes," congratulations! You are one of the few who are living true to themselves and their dreams.

If the answer is "no," then the next question is why not? Many will answer by describing obstacles such as not having enough money, being restricted by family obligations, experiencing an abusive childhood, or lacking adequate schooling, intelligence, or self-discipline. You might blame others or outside situations, or you might point a figure toward yourself with critical self-blame.

Forget all this blaming and ask yourself one empowering question: How can I express myself fully? Do one thing today that is genuinely authentic. Take even a small step; insist on being who you are. Prepare your favorite dinner for yourself, sign up for a class in which you are interested, put on that swirling skirt you love to feel dancing around your legs, soak in a bath surrounded by candlelight. Who's stopping you? No one at all.

Unroll Your Ears

God made all pleasures innocent.
—CAROLINE SHERIDAN NORTON, *The Lady of LaGaraye* (1862)

I always get a kick out of my clients' reactions to massaging their ears. Few of us have spent much time touching our ears, except perhaps for cleaning or nuzzling with our partner.

Ears, surprisingly, can carry a great deal of tension. Some practitioners believe the ear holds many acupressure points that can affect the entire body. All I know for sure is that most of my clients smile, some of them sigh, and all of them relax when I massage their ears.

Start your ear massage by taking off any earrings you might be wearing. That alone may help your ears feel better. Gently squeeze both ear lobes between your thumb and forefinger, rolling the lobe back and forth. Be careful not to pinch or bruise yourself.

Next, continue this rolling motion up the outside borders of your ears, along the sides to where your ears intersect with your head. Slowly work your way back down.

Place your forefinger inside your ear (but not inside the ear canal) and, with your thumb behind your ear, gently massage the skin and cartilage.

Lastly, place your forefinger directly behind your earlobe where your jaw and neck intersect. Slowly run your finger up the back of your ear, along the groove, spreading your ear away from your head. This will release tension and stimulate your immune system.

Speak Your Truth

I have bursts of being a lady, but it doesn't last long.
—SHELLY WINTERS, Actor

As a little girl, I heard the phrase, "If you don't have something nice to say, don't say anything at all." Wanting to be a lady, I tried to say only "nice" things, whether they were true or not.

I did not realize how rampant this way of thinking is among women until I began my body work practice. Even when I specifically ask, "How does this feel?" or "Does this hurt?" many of my clients tell me it is hard for them to be honest about how they feel or what they are experiencing. After years of aiming to please others, it can be hard to believe that anyone actually wants to know how they feel.

Even though we have been taught to be "ladies," our bodies are not so cooperative. A client may say, "No, that doesn't hurt," while her feet spasm away from my touch. Or I might hear, "Am I anxious? No, I feel fine," as my client's rib cage lies motionless because she's holding her breath. Whenever there is a contradiction between what a client says and what her body tells me, I've learned to believe the embodied rather than the spoken communication. Our bodies are not so polite as to lie.

If others in your life are observant, they will also notice the discrepancy between what you say and what your body reveals. So you might as well just tell the truth. Speak up when you're feeling pain, discomfort, anxiety, or any other un-nice emotion. Follow your body, which is fully female and yet fully truthful. You will be led out of the trap of being a lady and into the joyful experience of being an embodied woman.

Make Massages Not War

If women ruled the world and we all got massages,
there would be no war.
—CARRIE SNOW, Comedian

I don't know if there would be no war if women ruled the world, but I do suspect that if everyone on the planet, especially those in power, were getting regular massages, the world would be a more peaceful, less violent place. In fact, the amount of touch we receive, especially as children, heavily influences how emotionally healthy or physically violent we may become.

In one scientific study, baby monkeys were taken from their mothers and thereby deprived of natural, nurturing touch. While these infants had all their other needs met, their touch needs were completely ignored. When these baby monkeys grew into adults and had babies of their own, the researchers had to remove their babies from the cage to keep the touch-deprived mother monkeys from killing them. The lack of touch, even though all other needs were met, left these monkeys angry, dangerous, and unable to bond in protective ways with their own offspring.

Touch is critical for us to be kind, loving women. Share a massage with someone you love.

Stretch Your Pelvis

We cannot do everything at once, but we can do something at once.
—CALVIN COOLIDGE (1872-1933)

Take advantage of those moments you're watching your favorite shows by stretching your pelvis! Lie on your back and take a deep breath. Slowly bring your right knee up to your chest, wrap your arms around your knee, and feel the stretch in your hip muscles. Don't strain them; this is a stretch, a sensuous, relaxing stretch. After a minute or so, lower your right leg and repeat with the left. Move slowly and smoothly. Lower your left leg and then bring both knees up together, stretching both sides of your pelvic area at the same time. Wasn't that better than watching a commercial? (If you've had any back or joint problems consult with your doctor before doing this exercise; and of course, no one should continue if it causes any discomfort.)

Co-Create with God

When we nurture and delight in our body, when we use it for the good of humankind, we co-create with God.
—CARL KOCH AND JOYCE HEIL, *Created in God's Image* (1991)

A while back I was invited to speak at a large, hunger-relief organization conference. Apparently one of the conference organizers was not clear about the subject of my talk, because when I told him I was giving a presentation on making peace with our bodies, his face turned white. I smiled and said, "Trust me on this. This will turn out fine." He nodded his head but did not seem to be able to speak. After my presentation, he approached me with a big smile. "You were right," he said. "You have an important message. I just couldn't imagine what you could say that was appropriate about the body!"

So many in our society, even well-meaning people who care about others, are afraid of the body (as a topic) and their bodies (in particular). Were you taught to fear your body? I was. Consequently, I was cut off from God and my creativity in significant ways. If we live only in our mind and spirits, how can we make a difference in the material world? Without creating through our bodies we are unable to tend our gardens, rock our babies to sleep, or carve a sculpture. Without using our senses, we are unable to create new recipes, write music, or capture a loved one's image on film.

Be godlike today. Delight in your body and create, co-create, with God.

Binge on Life

Life itself is the proper binge.
—JULIA CHILD, Chef

Many of us who are at odds with our bodies are addicted in some way to food. I combine work addiction with eating too little. The more stress, the less connected I am with my body. The less connected I am with my body, the more stress I suffer. During these times, I rarely eat because I rarely feel hungry. My stomach is too upset with worry and stress.

I've found it's nearly impossible to force myself to eat. My stomach is upset because I'm overwhelmed, not because I'm undisciplined. I try not to blame myself but instead use my loss of appetite as a sign that things need to change. Perhaps I need to resign from one of the projects I'm working on, or take a long weekend to rest from a demanding week. I may have invited someone dangerous into my life, and my body is trying to warn me. Or maybe I need a nurturing massage to soothe and refresh my body and emotions.

Is there something in your life you can't quite digest? Let your body lead you to changes that need to be made.

Welcome Your Body

It is easier for us to speak of the "personality" as identical with
the self than it is to speak of the body and the self as one.
"I am a personality" simply sounds more natural than "I am a body."
—JAMES NELSON, *Embodiment* (1978)

Are you a body, or do you have a body?

Before my burnout in 1985, my body was a possession, an "it" with whom I was oftentimes waging war. I viewed my body as an unruly slave that got my attention only when it let me down.

I am learning that I and my body are on the same team. We are the same team. The more I view myself as a body, the healthier and happier I become.

How do you view your body? As you, or as an it? It is time to personalize your body and move it from being an object, your possession, and welcome your body as a part of your very self.

Celebrate Your Digestion

And it is well to eat slowly: The food seems to be more plentiful,
probably because it lasts longer.
—M.F.K. FISHER (1908-1992)

We need food to fuel our bodies' engines, a task our digestive tract is marvelously constructed to accomplish in an energy-efficient way. Carl Koch and Joyce Heil write in *Created in God's Image*, "To realize the effectiveness of our digestive system, consider this: the food energy contained in three ounces of carbohydrate (equivalent to about 1.4 ounces of gasoline) is enough to fuel someone to ride a bicycle for an hour at a speed of ten miles per hour. If our bodies used gasoline instead of food, we could ride over nine hundred miles on one gallon of gas. How's that for fuel efficiency?"

I'd say that's fairly efficient. Let's celebrate our miraculous digestive systems. List in your body journal all the reasons you appreciate your digestive system.

Insist on Safety

Saying no can be the ultimate in self-care.
—CLAUDIA BLACK, Psychologist

Fear is more than an uncomfortable emotion. It is the body's emphatic statement that we are important. So valuable are we, so significant is our survival, that if we are threatened in any way, our bodies automatically give us extra power to protect ourselves, setting off alarms in all of our systems—respiratory, cardiovascular, muscular, endocrine, lymphatic, digestive, even the urinary system. Fear celebrates our worth by insisting on bringing our full attention to our need for protection.

Let "no" be your reponse to a threat. A quiet, emphatic "no" to unsafe sex, an unspoken "no" when refusing to walk down a street that feels dangerous, an explosive "no" when confronted with increased danger.

Practice. Turn your combustible energy toward the threat. Shove the air out of your lungs, through your voice, and into the air, declaring your boundaries with "No, no, no!"

Then take a deep breath and let go, let go, let go of fear. Breathe deeply and say "yes" to safety.

Affirm Your Sexuality

Sexuality is a sacrament.
—STARHAWK, *The Spiral Dance* (1979)

Write in the numbers indicating how often, if ever, the statements are true. Modify those statements that don't apply to you. 1—Never, 2—Sometimes, 3—Always.

___I feel adept at relating sexually.

___I feel attractive and sexually appealing.

___I feel comfortable with my body when I express myself sexually.

___I have an accurate understanding of reproduction.

___My relationships with women affirm my femininity.

___My relationships with men affirm my femininity.

___I protect myself against sexually transmitted disease.

___I say "no" to intimate touch that feels uncomfortable.

___When sexual with my partner, I experience regular orgasm.

___I feel comfortable pleasuring myself and do so regularly.

___I discuss and resolve sexual issues with my partner.

___If my partner and I have extended sexual difficulty, we seek appropriate professional help in a timely manner.

___I discuss sexual concerns with women friends.

___I am clear and comfortable about my sexual orientation.

___I regularly receive massage to meet my need for touch.

Scoring Evaluation

37-45   Congratulations! You are comfortable sexually.

26-36   Watch out. You aren't fully enjoying your sexual potential.

0-25   Body alert! Pay attention to your sexual needs.

Decrease Your Chances of Breast Cancer

Currently, one in nine (some studies say one in eight) women in the United States between the ages of one and eighty-five years gets breast cancer. This does not mean that one in nine forty-five-year-old women will get it. But breast cancer is the leading cause of death among American women who are forty to fifty-five years of age.
—CHRISTIANE NORTHRUP, M.D., *Women's Bodies,*
Women's Wisdom (1994)

I *found a lump.*
These words strike fear into the heart of every woman I know. While there is no guaranteed way to prevent breast cancer, some studies have suggested that there are a few things we can do to lower our chances of contracting this disease.

First, cut back on your fat intake. Stay away from the juicy steaks, the buttery desserts, and the whole milk products.

Second, keep your weight at a healthy level. If you're cutting out the fat anyway, your weight will probably drop as well.

Third, drink less alcohol, no more than two drinks per week. Some studies have shown that women who drink three or more alcoholic beverages a week have an increased chance of contracting breast cancer.

Fourth, give yourself monthly breast exams and get mammograms with the regularity that your doctor suggests. In the event that cancer does occur, early detection can save your life. Your life is worth saving.

SEPTEMBER

WORD WRAP

I want to wrap words
like a soft terry cloth robe
around my flawed nakedness
to comfort my shame
with cover.

But words
cannot be pulled
off a bathroom hook
or made to drape and enfold
chilled flesh.

So
my humanness
will remain
betrayed.

Recognize Your Body Pattern

*All sanity depends on this: that it should be a delight to feel heat
strike the skin, a delight to stand upright, knowing the bones are
moving easily under the flesh.*
—DORIS LESSING

My father recently put our home movies onto video. One of my favorite segments was a family gathering in the backyard of my childhood home, with me and my dog, Poochie, running and playing around the feet of the grownups. How free I was with my body at that time. My long auburn hair blew behind me as Poochie and I wrestled, chased, and played without a self-conscious thought in the world. I couldn't help but notice how differently I move now, more cautiously, more fearful of criticism.

Our bodies record our experiences from conception through death. We now know that even in the womb, babies respond to noises, lights, movement, and other environmental factors affecting their development, including their posture and movements. Once out of the womb, external factors continue to shape our bodies. If we are well cared for, our bodies will stand upright, our skin will welcome touch, our eyes will take in all the glories around us. All of our senses will be alive to living, and we will live well.

If, however, our needs are neglected or we experience trauma, our bodies will be negatively affected. Carolyn Braddock, in her book *Body Voices*, describes three ways women who have been traumatized may hold their bodies—rigid, collapsed, and inanimate.

Women with rigid body patterns present a strong front to the world, with hands and jaws clenched, shoulders high, and breathing shallow. These women hide their vulnerability under an armored body, hoping that they will avoid being hurt again.

Those who feel defeated may wear a collapsed body pattern, with head hung down, shoulders slumped, and breath weak. Hoping to be overlooked, these women shrink back from confrontation. Depression and a sense of powerlessness is common for women in this pattern.

The inanimate woman seems to float above her body, feet barely connected to the ground and a distant look in her eyes. This body pattern (my personal favorite) works under the misguided impression that pain can be avoided if the body is avoided.

Sadly, none of these patterns resolves past pain, or serves as an effective way to protect the self from present danger.

What does your body tell you about the past? Do you recognize yourself in any of these three descriptions? You might want to discuss these body patterns with your body buddy or support group. Ask for feedback on how they see you carrying yourself and your pain. Listen to your body, for there is truth inside your tissues, truth that if acknowledged will set you free.

Return to Feelgoodallover

Do not wish to be anything but what you are,
and try to be that perfectly.
—St. Francis de Sales

Ready to take another trip to Feelgoodallover? Grab the list of things that make you feel good about yourself which you made on your first trip on April 8th. Find a blank audio cassette and pop it into your tape recorder. In your clearest, most enthusiastic, energetic Feelgoodallover voice, read your list into the microphone. A few minutes later, you have your very own Feelgoodallover tape! Ta da!

Now, whether you spend time at home or are on the move, you can listen to your tape. You will hear yourself declare all the reasons you have for feeling great about yourself. Listen to yourself listing all of the people who make your life special. The support you get from your sister, the wisdom your grandfather offers, the spontaneous, humorous phone calls you receive from your best buddy. You smile as you think about a romantic interest and the private moments you share (or will share). Just thinking about these people makes you feel good all over.

You settle into a feeling of competence and contentment as you remind yourself of the qualities of which you may be proud. Your intelligence, your stamina, your courage, your kindness. You remember the parts of your body you admire, the softness of your hair, the color of your eyes, the strength in your hands, the smoothness of your thighs.

Welcome back. You are once again in the land of Feelgoodallover.

Change Your Feelings by Changing Your Body

The body is like a river of information and energy, we are learning,
and all its parts have a dynamic communication
with all the other parts.
—CHRISTIANE NORTHRUP, M.D., *Women's Bodies,*
Women's Wisdom (1994)

Last summer the air conditioner went out in my car during one of the heat waves common in southern California. With sweat dripping down my back and my blouse stuck to the car seat, all I wanted to do was get home quickly. Unfortunately, a traffic jam forced me to merely inch along in the searing heat.

When I finally reached the door, I was irrationally irritated, muttering at my keys for not opening the door sooner. Once inside, I threw my purse on the floor, stripped off my blouse, and headed straight for the refrigerator. After a few moments of sticking my head in the freezer, I had cooled down enough to regain some semblance of sanity, and I made myself a tall, cool pitcher of water with sliced lemon and cucumber.

In a few moments I had gone from a wild woman on the road to a relaxed, rational being stretched out on my couch, stroking my cats. How did I make that transformation? Through attending to my body. Lowering my body temperature through drinking a cool drink, removing some clothing, and breathing the cool air of my freezer not only made my body feel better but radically altered my emotional state.

When you find yourself irritable, try changing your body's state, either by raising or lowering your temperature, by drinking something hot or cold, or by changing positions. Often, changing some aspect of your physical self will affect your emotional self.

Celebrate Your Hands

The hands are one of the most complex structures in our body: of the 30 bones in the whole arm, 27 are to be found in the hand, making it particularly susceptible to stress and tension. The good news is that they are exquisitely sensitive, and love being massaged.
—ROBERT THÉ, *5-Minute Massage* (1995)

Let's thank our hands by treating them to a sensual massage. You'll need massage oil, a tape of relaxing music and a tape player, a large pitcher filled with ice water garnished with strawberries, and a small towel. Invite a friend, or enjoy this hand celebration on your own.

Turn on a tape of relaxing music, imagining the delights of a European spa are yours. A beautiful woman (or man, depending on your fantasy) leads you to a cozy place to relax, offering you a glass of spa water. The chill awakens your mouth.

Stretch your fingers in the air for a few moments, noticing how they feel. Squeeze the bottle of massage oil slightly to let the fragrance waft toward your nose. Let your breath grow deeper.

Pour oil into your palm and rub your hands together to warm the oil. Rub your right hand around your left wrist. Cover the top of your hand with oil, and then reach underneath and soothe your palm as well. Concentrate on the parts that feel sore, slowly massaging the tension from your left hand. Taking each finger in turn, caress under, around, and over each digit.

Eventually, move to the other hand. Soothing out the pains, tell your hands how grateful you are for accomplishing a myriad of tasks everyday. Promise not to take them for granted in the future. Take another sip of water, noticing the delicious flavor. Breathe slowly in and out. Visit your personal spa regularly.

Assess Your Stress

There is less leisure now than in the Middle Ages, when one-third of the year consisted of holidays and festivals.
—RALPH BORSODI

In an international study, researchers found that Americans have the least amount of vacation time of all industrialized nations. Did you get your share of vacation time this summer? Is your life stressful these days or rather calm?

Let's find out by asking your body. Pull out your body journal and draw an outline of your body. Color in the stressed places. Be careful to mark all the areas that feel tight or out of whack. Got an upset stomach? How about a twitch in your left eye? Are your thighs aching? These could be signs of stress.

Compare today's drawing with those you've created in the past. What areas of your body are most often affected? Ask your body if you need a vacation. If you've had a vacation, did you structure it so your body could relax? Assess your stress post-vacation as well. Discuss your pictures with your support group, body buddy, or a friend who supports your body's need for rest and recuperation.

Be Powerful

There are two kinds of women: those who want power in the world,
and those who want power in bed.
—JACQUELINE KENNEDY ONASSIS (1929-1994)

Many women believe personal power is derived from relationships with men. Either we please men, becoming wives, lovers, and nurturers, or we compete with men, becoming colleagues and business associates. I believe as long as we hang our sense of power on masculine relationships, we will continue to feel bad about ourselves and our bodies. How can we not, when we've given men so much control over assessing our performance in both the bedroom and the boardroom?

Feminine power is a profoundly potent but too often untapped resource for today's woman. We discover feminine strength, not in relationships with men, but in relationships with women and our own bodies. We learn how to be strong women from other strong women, and from the wisdom and flesh-and-blood instincts offered by a deep connection with our bodies. Some believe that masculine energy moves down through the body and to the earth, and that feminine energy draws power from the earth, swirling up through the body and out through the voice.

Be powerful in your own body. Take off your shoes and let your feet feel the earth. Draw energy from the feminine, from your female body, the physical source of power.

Rotate Your Ankles

*Our legs and feet are probably the hardest working and most
neglected parts of our bodies. . . . As anyone who has had a sprained
or twisted ankle can confirm, the ankle is a very important part of
our body: a small, flexible region which connects the foot
with the rest of the body, and acts as a shock absorber,
supporting our entire weight.*
—ROBERT THÉ, *5-Minute Massage* (1995)

When I'm working on a book project, I usually write in eight
to ten-hour blocks of time. That's a lot of sitting, which my
body doesn't enjoy. After a few hours, I'll find myself squirming in
my chair, trying to get comfortable, as my back, shoulders, legs,
and feet begin to complain.

One way I keep my feet happy is to stop every so often and
rotate my ankles. It always amazes me how simply moving one foot
and then the other slowly in a circular motion can refresh the rest
of my body. Rotating your ankles encourages circulation in your
feet, calves, and even upper legs. Breathing along with the rotation
exercise helps relax my upper body as well. And focusing attention
on my ankles, even for a few moments, helps me let go of the intense
concentration needed to write and relaxes my brain. A few rotations
on each ankle and I'm refreshed and ready to start again.

Try this next time you sit for long periods of time at work, in a
car, while flying, or while waiting for someone to arrive. You'll
remind yourself of your need to be grounded in your body, and
your whole self will benefit.

Exhale Fear, Inhale Courage

I define self-nurturance as having the courage
to pay attention to your needs.
—JENNIFER LOUDEN, *The Woman's Comfort Book* (1992)

I eased myself down onto the massage table, my head still buzzing with the day's activities. When I felt the massage therapist's hands gently touch my shoulders, tears stung my eyes and my throat tightened. A jolt of fear zig-zagged through my body.

I took a deep breath and asked myself, "What does this mean?" The phrase went through my mind, "You are afraid."

"Of what?" I took a few more deep breaths, clearing my head of the buzz, waiting to hear the answer. After a few moments, I knew.

I was afraid of resting. I asked myself an open-ended question: "What will happen if I rest?"

In rhythm with my breath, I answered the question:

"If I rest, I'll be selfish."

"If I rest, I'll waste time."

"If I rest, I'll fail financially."

"If I rest, I'll let my friends down."

"If I rest, I'll never get up again."

Loving our bodies is a courageous act. Listening to our bodies' wisdom is an activity that invokes all the "rules" we've unknowingly adopted that reject self-care. The path you and I share is not one that many women around us travel. Sometimes being on a different path can feel scary.

Take a deep breath, drawing the air down into your toes. Inhale courage. Exhale fear. Inhale courage. Exhale fear. Continue this exercise for several minutes until your body and your courage are refreshed and vital.

Tune Out with Tea

Tea quenches tears and thirst.
—JEANINE LARMOTH AND CHARLOTTE TURGEON,
Murder on the Menu (1972)

Let tea soothe your soul and reduce the bags under your eyes. Make a big pitcher of chamomile iced tea and pour yourself a tall, cool glass. After taking a few sips, collect six of the used tea bags (cool them off in the fridge first). Play some soothing music and stretch out on the sofa. Place the tea bags over and around your eyes, covering your eyelids and the skin surrounding your eye area. The coolness and the tea will help reduce puffiness, soothe tired eyes, and help you look and feel more alive. Tune out with tea, a great remedy for a rough day.

Locate Anger in Your Body

Anger is a signal, and one worth listening to.
—HARRIET LERNER, *The Dance of Anger* (1985)

One of my clients recently told me, "I'm so angry I feel like I could burst!" and then she did. A torrent of tears spilled down her cheeks as she described a hurtful conversation she had just had with a close friend. As I listened to her words, I also paid careful attention to how her body was expressing her rage. She gasped for breath in-between sobs. One of her legs curled underneath her as her hands rolled into fists and unrolled. In addition to what I could observe, I suspect that she was experiencing her body's rage through her heart rate, tension in her abdomen, and other internal changes.

How does your body communicate anger? What parts of your body grow tense or relaxed? What physical changes do you experience when you get angry and when you calm down? Do your pulse and breath quicken? Does your jaw clench or your stomach churn? Do you break out in a rash? Feel pain in your scalp? Take time to locate anger in your body and record this information in your body journal. You may describe how your body feels anger, or you may draw an outline of your body and color in the angry places. Whatever format works best for you is the one to use. Anger is an important and potentially dangerous emotion, an emotion your body can help you better understand and express in helpful ways.

Celebrate Your Beauty

To seek after beauty as an end, is a wild goose chase, a will-o'-the-wisp, because it is to misunderstand the very nature of beauty, which is the normal condition of a thing being as it should be.
—ADE BETHUNE, in JUDITH STOUGHTON,
Proud Donkey of Schaerbeek (1988)

What is beauty? The answer to this question depends on the person asked. Cross-cultural studies illustrate that women's beauty is defined differently by different cultures. The Japanese find the back of the neck especially appealing, while Western cultures focus attention on breast size. Often beauty is linked with signs of wealth. For some, being thin is attractive because it implies the woman (or her husband) is wealthy enough to support her leisure time to tan, exercise, and relax. In other cultures, larger women are considered beautiful because weight implies the wealth needed to have plenty to eat without physical labor.

In order to make peace with our bodies, we cannot simply accept the definitions of beauty given to us by our society, because these standards are arbitrary and impossible to meet. Rather than accept someone else's definition of beauty, take time today and ponder what beauty truly is to you. Have you already achieved it?

Act Confident

It is best in the theater to act with confidence no matter
how little right you have to it.
—LILLIAN HELLMAN (1907-1984)

Years ago I interviewed convicted sex offenders and asked them how they selected the children they molested. Time and time again, the answer was the same, "We look for those who are lonely, the good kids, the ones who won't resist."

Whether a sex offender is targeting a child or an adult woman, these predators look for someone they can overpower, intimidate, and exploit. They often watch for body language that reflects powerlessness, weakness, and vulnerability.

While no technique is foolproof, experts in criminal behavior recommend presenting yourself as a woman with confidence, someone who is willing and able to put up resistance. When you are out, walk with a strong gait, eyes open and aware of your surroundings. Hold your head up and your shoulders back. You may be scared down to your toes, but exhibiting an air of power may convince a would-be attacker that you are a woman he'd be a fool to bother.

Be Absorbed in Pleasure

If you let yourself be absorbed completely, if you surrender completely to the moments as they pass, you live more richly those moments.
—ANNE MORROW LINDBERGH, *Bring Me a Unicorn* (1971)

Ever throw a party you hoped would be fun, but got so caught up in the details and in making sure everyone else was having a good time, that you were uptight during the shindig and exhausted afterward?

I've done this too many times. Each year I co-host an annual Pumpkin Pie Party where about fifty to seventy-five people come together and make pumpkin pies from scratch. We have a pumpkin carving contest, eats lots of wonderful food, and have a great time. Or I should say, I'm *learning* to have a great time. Each year, as I grow more determined that my body attend the party too, I take some of the pressure off myself. I do things a little simpler, take a little less responsibility for other people's happiness, and pay more attention to my own enjoyment. The less I'm concerned about detail, and the more I simply become a partygoer, the better time I have.

How can you release yourself from anxiety-producing attitudes and focusing on the needs of others so that you can become absorbed in the pleasure of the moment?

Forgive Yourself

You may have to fight a battle more than once to win it.
—Margaret Thatcher, Former British Prime Minister

Do you know how many times I've started an exercise program? Me neither. I've lost count.

I begin an exercise plan and last a few days, get distracted (by anything and everything), and the next thing I know it's a week later and I haven't exercised again. How did that happen?

And so I forgive myself for breaking a promise to myself and start again. And again. And again. I may not be perfect, but at least I'm persistent. And maybe I'll have to content myself with that victory—that I keep on trying, even if I haven't mastered this particular aspect of my life.

Do you have something in your life that makes you feel like a failure? We all do. So, join the club. Today, give yourself a break. When the little voice nags at you, nag back. Make a list in your body journal of all the things you like about yourself. The better you feel about yourself, the more likely you'll follow through on promises you make yourself. The more you heap guilt, shame, and blame on yourself, the less you will like yourself, and the more you will resist caring for yourself. Tell that nagging voice to listen while you read aloud all the great things about you. This approach has helped me turn that exercise tape on one more time rather than flop on the couch in self-loathing despair.

Show Your Soul

The heart is only one of the many organs out of whose functions and shapes metaphoric richness has appeared over time. Historically, soul is to be found in the spleen, the liver, the stomach, the gall bladder, the intestines, the pituitary, and the lungs. . . . Is this mere poetic license, or is it the power of the body in its many varied parts to create a polycentric field for the soul?
—THOMAS MOORE, *Care of the Soul* (1992)

I remember as a young schoolgirl standing with my classmates each morning and placing my hand over my heart. Together our young voices would pledge allegiance to the "flag of the United States of America." Simply saying the words of the pledge was not really saying it. We needed to be standing with our hands over our hearts for the pledge to be real.

Allegiance to a country, a person, or a spiritual path requires more than lip service. Our bodies and our souls must join together to illustrate our passion and commitment. We are urged by prophets to "love the Lord your God with all your heart and with all your soul and with all your might." The rest of your body is also welcome into this love relationship. Love God with your feet by being grounded physically and spiritually; with your hands as you touch others with nurturing kindness; with your smile as you enjoy the fragrance of a rose; with your very breath as you meditate on God's love.

Let your entire body participate in your spiritual journey. An inner awareness of God's presence may be a beginning point, but must culminate in action to be complete. Show your soul by the way you treat your body and in your body's actions.

Let Go of Blame

Take your life in your own hands and what happens?
A terrible thing: no one to blame.
—Erica Jong

When I was a little girl, I fell out of a tree and dislocated my right elbow. My parents rushed me to the doctor, who neglected to X-ray my arm and misdiagnosed the injury as a sprain. Not until years later did we realize that my arm did not fully extend due to the fact that the dislocated bone had pinched my bicep nerve, permanently damaging the development of that muscle.

Who's to blame for my disability? No one. The doctor misdiagnosed my injury, but spending time being angry at him now will not bring my bicep back to its potential. Instead, ruminating on how victimized I am further disempowers me.

The empowering question to ask is, "Who's responsible?" And the answer is, "I am." Although not responsible for the original problem, I am responsible for building up my muscles to the extent they are now capable, making sure that I have the strength I need to carry on my life and continue my massage and body work practice. It is my responsibility to confront my feelings of insecurity that come from having one arm that looks different from the other. It's up to me to take what I've been given and create the most loving, vital life possible, and that task requires all my time and energy. Wasting even a moment blaming someone else takes me off-course.

Are you wasting your valuable time and energy blaming someone else for something that has negatively affected your body? Turn that blame into power by taking responsibility for your present life. Come home to your body by letting go of the blame.

Endure Wisdom

Endurance is only the beginning. There must be acceptance and the knowledge that sorrow fully accepted brings its own gifts. For there is alchemy in sorrow. It can be transmuted into wisdom.
—PEARL S. BUCK, *The Child Who Never Grew* (1950)

A close friend described to me the terror of finding an intruder in her home as she returned from her morning run. Because he ran from the house at the sound of her approach, the story had a safe ending. But my stomach soured as I was reminded that she might have been taken from me, in an instant, and there was nothing I could have done to prevent this tragic loss.

I hate acknowledging the limits of my power, enduring the reality that I and those I love will not be on this earth forever. I can't change the fact that my body is aging and my hair is turning gray. I can't change the fact that after years of wear and tear, my teeth crack. Nor can I turn hot fudge sundaes, burritos, or cheese-covered tortillas into food that helps my arteries work better.

While it is important to improve those areas over which we have control, today focus attention on those areas that are beyond human power. As you struggle with the fear, anger, resistance, and sadness that flows from facing limitations, a sense of wisdom will emerge. Wisdom is not knowledge, but a restful resignation to what is and what will never be.

Celebrate Your Sense of Smell

Nothing is more memorable than a scent.
—DIANE ACKERMAN, *A Natural History of the Senses* (1990)

I walk into the massage room and fill my nostrils with the scents of nurturance—the smell of fresh sheets and lavender-scented oil. Before the massage therapist touches me, my muscles are already starting to relax, signaled by the aromas I know so well. My body knows what these fragrances mean—tenderness, soothing touch, rejuvenation.

Celebrate your nose today by writing in your body journal the scents you find pleasurable. Perhaps you love the smell of gardenias. Or the scent of a freshly bathed baby. Does the aroma of bread baking in the oven fill you with anticipation? Or the smell of freshly mowed grass on a warm fall afternoon? Consciously bring one of your "pleasure scents" into your life today.

Be a Little Pushy

As women, we are taught to meet everyone else's needs before we nurture ourselves. And as we are groomed into compliant beings, we come to believe that the people in our lives will anticipate and meet our needs as we do theirs. When this does not happen, we begin to feel we do not have a right to our needs and desires.
—JENNIFER LOUDEN, *The Woman's Comfort Book* (1992)

Ever been told you're too loud or too aggressive? Sometimes we're put in small, quiet boxes and told to behave. The general attitude assumes men are the sole culprits for this repressive pressure. However, we women may also act disapproving of other females who speak their mind or appear a bit too pushy. According to a recent study from the University of Minnesota, female managers were more likely to hire timid, self-effacing women than were their male counterparts. Apparently, we women are more attracted to working with "team players."

Whether men or other women reward us for ignoring our individuality, we have a right to our feelings, sensations, and longings. While no one has the right to violate someone else's boundaries, none of us is obligated to meet the expectations of others. Just ask your body, "What do I need?"

Do you need time off? Push for a vacation.

Do you need money for massages? Push for a raise.

Do you need time alone? Push for help with the kids.

Do you need exercise? Push for dance lessons.

Do you need sunshine? Push for a day at the beach.

Let your body help you decide what you need and when to push.

Reject Rejection

Creative minds have always been known
to survive any kind of bad training.
—ANNA FREUD (1895-1982)

I went to the grocery store to get cereal, milk, and cat food. What I came home with was a little more self-hatred. Innocently, I stood at the checkout counter, desiring nothing more than to pay for my items. But what was available to me, free of charge, was a bombardment of images of how I'm supposed to look, as illustrated by women on the magazine covers. Thin, smooth thighs and soft, perky breasts let me know I was inferior. Clear faces with no wrinkles around their eyes told me I was too old.

Whether you've suffered direct abuse or not, every woman in this society has been given negative and destructive messages about her body. We must protect ourselves from these images, replacing them with kind, realistic statements of womanhood.

Pay attention to the many ways, spoken and visual, you are told today that your body is unacceptable. Jot these down in your body journal. Maybe someone makes a joke about the size of your feet or the shape of your ears. A TV ad may advise you that your teeth aren't white enough. A magazine image may inform you that your skin is not tan enough or your biceps firm enough. Make a full list.

Next to each criticism, write a positive statement about your body. Assert that your feet are just the right size to get where you need to go; your ears can hear clearly; your teeth are strong; your skin is smooth; your biceps are strong enough to close the door to unwanted critiques. Apply your vast, feminine creative powers to rejecting these false and hurtful messages.

Eat When You're Hungry

It is not immoral not to finish a meal, but it is of questionable morality to treat yourself like a waste-disposal system.
—JANE BRODY

When I was a young girl, Allen Sherman was a popular comedian who said his mother always told him to clean his plate because the children in Europe were starving. So he cleaned his plate. The problem was that the children in Europe kept starving and he gained weight.

Depending upon how old you are (and what particular nation was experiencing the most devastation) you may have heard your parents say something like, "Eat your dinner, the children in Europe (Korea, Bangladesh, Biafra, China, Bosnia) are starving." Or you may have been made to feel that not cleaning your plate indicated that you didn't appreciate your mother or other caretaker.

Many of us were fed a mixture of guilt along with our mashed potatoes and gravy, somehow linking our eating habits with the woes of the world or our level of appreciation for the food provider. To this day, the sight of a partially eaten meal, even if we have eaten our fill, may trigger a sense of guilt that has no basis in our present reality. While wasting food isn't to be condoned, overeating in the belief that somehow it helps some unfortunate child across the sea or expresses your affection is sheer folly.

It's time to separate a sense of compassion for the hungry from your own eating patterns. Genuinely help the hungry by writing a check to a local or world hunger relief organization. Show your affection for your mother in some other way, such as going for a walk with her. And feel content when you stop eating whenever your stomach is full.

Honor Your Body as a Spiritual Temple

Do you not know that your body is the temple of the Holy Spirit. . . .
Therefore honor God with your body.
—I CORINTHIANS 6:19, 20, *New American Standard Bible*

Many of us have been raised, or at least influenced, by religious traditions that degrade the body. Christian theology has long blamed "the flesh" for all unacceptable behaviors. Eastern religions have urged us to "transcend" our bodies and all desire by ignoring or not even experiencing our bodily needs. Few traditional organized religions give the body the respect it deserves.

Conversely, in a drastic reactionary swing against a negative view of the body, some in our society all but worship the body through various sacraments. Some are devoted to the god of nutrition, meticulously counting fat grams. Others bow to the hard-body god, working their muscles into knots of steel. Recruiting new converts, diet deities make the talk show circuit touting their particular eating rituals.

Somewhere in the midst of these extremes, factions, and dogmas is a simple truth: Our bodies are made in the image of God and are therefore precious beyond gold, wise beyond measure, and worthy of our respect and care. Your body is the creation of God. Honor your body as your spiritual temple.

Be Selfish

*Putting oneself down is narcissism in reverse. . . . The healing of
narcissism, the fulfillment of its symptomatic hunger, is achieved by
giving the ego what it needs—pleasure in accomplishment,
acceptance, and some degree of recognition. . . . The secret to healing
narcissism is not to heal it at all, but to listen to it.*
—THOMAS MOORE, *Care of the Soul* (1992)

A client told me, "You've really helped me."
"Oh, it was nothing," I replied as a piercing pain shot through
my shoulder and upper arm. I ignored it, hoping it would go away
on its own. It didn't. Later that day when the pain became unbearable, I listened. Lying on my back, I raised my arm slowly and
asked myself, "What does this mean?"

"Say thank you." came the reply.

"What?" I asked the blazing red pain in my shoulder.

"Say thank you," my shoulder said. "Why do you degrade your
contribution to others? You nurture them through body work and
they nurture you through appreciation. Receive it."

"But it feels so selfish," I responded.

"Then be selfish," my shoulder said.

My shoulder carried the pain of an unloved self while I was
worried about becoming too conceited. Tout your accomplishments,
beat your drum, toot your horn! You deserve all the accolades you
can get. If you're depriving yourself of the nurturance you need,
you may have a pain or a twinge that will speak wisdom like my
shoulder spoke to me.

Look Before You Throw

Be careful of what you throw away.
—ELEANOR MCMILLEN BROWN

I have a friend who didn't get what she needed as a little girl. She grew up believing that she didn't deserve nice things and would feel guilty whenever she was given something special. In bouts of self-loathing, she would bag up many of her clothes, favorite books, her most comfortable chair, and other treasures and take them to thrift stores. This self-inflicted loss was motivated, not because she could no longer use these items, but because she felt she no longer deserved them.

It's been a joy watching her change over time as she has continued to be nurtured through therapy and body work. Rarely now does she deprive herself of beauty or comfort in response to unfounded feelings of shame and guilt. She is learning to receive more and benefit from what she receives.

Before you throw away something, question your motive. If you are genuinely finished with the item, then it is time to let go. But be careful to watch for a hidden desire to deprive yourself of good things. Good things are good! So let yourself (and your body) enjoy them.

Celebrate Mischief

I can sometimes resist temptation, but never mischief.
—JOYCE REBETA-BURDITT, *The Cracker Factory* (1977)

Have you been just a little too good lately? I thought so. Time to celebrate the wild woman inside you.

Grab your body buddy and get ready for a wild night on the town. Dress up in a "look" you've always admired, but never had the courage to pull off. You may want to start with wigs. Maybe you're a brunette who's always wanted to be a blonde. Or a blonde who's wanted to have a long, dark mane like Cher.

Then put on outfits you've always wanted to wear but would never show anyone you know. Hats, plumes, tight jeans, low-cut dresses, whatever suits your fantasy.

Once you're both all dolled up, drive to the next town (to avoid meeting anyone you know) and go dancing. If either of you are married, leave your partners at home just for tonight. Promise each other that you won't let the other go home with anyone (this is supposed to be fun, not dangerous). And then have a ball.

You'll come home refreshed, reconvinced of your desirability, more in love with your body, and ready to be good again.

Protect Your Home

*Of all the threats to the security of your home, the most common is
the residential burglar. The odds of your experiencing someone
invading the sanctity of your home, seizing part of or all
of your possessions and vanishing without a trace
are increasing dramatically each year.*
—HOWARD JONES, *Total Home Security* (1979)

Some dream theorists say that when we dream about our homes,
we are symbolizing our own bodies and how we view ourselves.
Certainly our homes are an extension of our personal boundaries
in which we house and protect our belongings, express our
personalities through decorating, and sleep at night expecting safety
for ourselves and loved ones.

Having someone break into our homes feels similar to having
our bodily space violated. We shudder at the thought of a stranger
being inside our space, as if burglary were another form of rape.

To better protect your home, consider these suggestions:

♦ Get a dog: You're ten times more likely to be burglarized if
you live in a house without a dog.

♦ Keep your door light burning: You're twice as likely to be
burglarized if your front door is dark.

♦ Install a burglar alarm: You're thirteen times less likely to be
burglarized if you have an alarm in working order.

Manage Your Emotions

. . . [O]ne of the few things human beings have to offer is the richness
of unconscious and conscious emotional responses to being alive.
—NTOZAKE SHANGE, in CLAUDIA TATE, ED.,
Black Women Writers at Work (1983)

Write in the numbers indicating how often, if ever, the statements are true. Modify those statements that don't apply to you. 1—Never, 2—Sometimes, 3—Always.

___I explore how my emotional life contributes to illness.

___I have a clear sense of what I need.

___I feel comfortable expressing my feelings to others.

___I am aware of places my body carries unexpressed emotion.

___I feel good about my body, even though it isn't "perfect."

___I take responsibility for managing my emotions.

___I rarely try to manage or control other people's emotions.

___I actively work to improve my opinion of my body.

___I take good care of my body.

___I respect the feelings of others.

___I do not allow people in my life who degrade my body.

___I have enthusiasm and energy for my life.

___I rarely feel depressed.

___I am resolving any past abuse that undermines emotional health.

___I regularly receive massage to facilitate emotional healing.

Scoring Evaluation

37-45   Great! Your emotions are managed well.

26-36   Watch out. Pay more attention to your emotions.

0-25   Body alert! Unexpressed emotions may undermine health.

Be Active, Be Rested

Night brings our troubles to the light, rather than banishes them.
—LUCIUS ANNAEUS SENECA (circa 4 B.C.-65 A.D.)

Having trouble sleeping at night because you're worrying about your problems?

I do from time to time and have learned a great deal about sleeping from my cats. Have you ever seen cats sleep? They curl in luxurious positions, with toes stretched and tails draped gracefully. These creatures are so connected to their bodies, they've turned a simple nap into a sensuous experience.

I believe their secret to sound sleep is their activity when they are awake. In-between snoozes, my cats dash all over the house, chasing each other, batting balls around the kitchen floor, climbing up the bookshelves to see how many books they can knock to the floor, and exploring cabinets I accidentally left ajar. They're alive, interested, and active.

The next thing I know, they're both sound asleep, looking more content than I ever hope to be. Take a lesson from the beasts, who have never learned how to disregard their bodies.

Be alive. Be interested. Be active. When it's time to sleep, your body will be more ready to relax and get the rest you need.

Walk a Prayer

Walking, I learned, is a kind of prayer, the body swinging alone at a steady rhythm as the legs and feet dance ever onwards and the soul is released.
—MICHELE ROBERTS

Prayer can be a powerful avenue of physical healing and disease prevention. Even the medical community, not traditionally known for its spiritual emphasis, is acknowledging the role of spirituality in health and healing. For example:

◆ Heart surgery patients with no religious beliefs in a 1995 Dartmouth-Hitcock Medical Center study were three times more likely to die than those who drew strength from their faith.

◆ Prayer is credited with helping female patients recovering from hip fractures walk farther when discharged and experience less depression than those in the study who drew little or no strength from their faith.

◆ Studies have shown that prayer can help insomniacs fall asleep (seventy-five percent of test group), infertile women become pregnant (thirty-five percent), and those with chronic pain rely on fewer pain medications (thirty-four percent).

Traditionally, prayer has been embodied in a kneeling position, our eyes looking downward in reverence before God. But prayer can also take on the bodily form of movement, with our eyes surveying the landscape in gratitude for the beauties of creation.

Walk your prayer today. Don't worry about putting your thoughts, longings, and feelings into words. Let your body say all you want to tell God with the free, open movement of your hands, the powerful stride of your legs, your lungs pulling in fresh air, and your eyes paying attention, filled with gratitude at what they see.

Be Imperfect

The sin of perfectionism is that it mutilates life
by demanding the impossible.
—JEROME FRANK

Life is too short to waste it trying to be perfect. You'll never achieve this goal, and you'll waste whatever time you have to enjoy this existence. Instead of setting your sights on perfection, try to be the best imperfect person you can be.

Set a goal of being imperfect: Enjoy wearing attractive, imperfect clothing over your fine, imperfect body. Style your imperfect hair around your beautiful though imperfect face. Continue with your imperfect exercise program, toning your imperfect muscles, and don't bother trying to achieve any unobtainable ideal. Isn't this fun? Deciding to achieve imperfection allows you to reach your goal and let go of unrealistic expectations.

OCTOBER

SIBILANT AND SENSELESS

Senses understimulated
with sights, sounds
and soothing strokes
in sensitive years
left synapses sluggish.

Subsequently, messages sent now
slide slowly along smooth sheaths
as scrambled, scattered signals,
creating subtle senselessness
and unsought solitude.

And so it is
that somewhat deaf
and sometimes blind
I sadly search the silent shadows
for simple signs of you.

Adopt the Motto "No pain? A lot gained"

Touch is ten times stronger than verbal or visual contact.
—SAUL SCHANBERG, Duke University

A client said, "The massage felt great, but I feel guilty about not accomplishing anything. Shouldn't I be working harder?"

The Puritan work ethic distorts our thinking about the benefits of pleasurable touch. We assume that if we receive rather than give, accept rather than act, we aren't doing anything. What about the adage "no pain, no gain"?

Actually, you can actively build your self-esteem while lying on a massage table. Research supports this claim. Dr. Sandra Weiss, a nurse and researcher, found that children with the highest self-esteem were those with the highest body awareness. They had a sense of, and were comfortable with, their bodies.

Researchers discovered that positive body awareness was created through the touch received regularly from their parents, touch characterized as comfortable, covering a large extent of their bodies, and intense enough to get their attention.

Comfortable touch: The children accepted their bodies because their parents touched them in safe, loving ways. Feeling lovable comes easily if your parents lovingly held you on their laps to comfort you or cuddle with you. The children welcomed and enjoyed this touch.

Extensive touch: Touch was not only comfortable, but also freely shared and abundantly available. Receiving more than just a pat on the head or an occasional hug, these children received non-invasive touch on their arms, legs, backs, and other nonsexual parts of their bodies.

Intense touch. Touch was intense enough to gain the child's attention. The parents wrestled with, hugged, walked hand-in-hand with, and massaged their children to communicate affection.

Did you receive this kind of touch when you were a child? If not, it isn't too late. These three characteristics of touch are those available through professional massage!

First, a professional massage is comfortable and soothing. Your skin is nourished, your circulation stimulated, and your immune system strengthened. Remember, it is illegal for a massage therapist to touch you in an erotic way. An important component in feeling comfortable with a massage therapist is knowing that he or she will honor your private boundaries. The goal is for you to receive a massage that is pleasurable, safe, and nurturing.

Second, you receive nurturing touch over a large extent of your body during a professional massage. My clients enjoy touch on parts of their bodies ordinarily left unattended, such as their calves, their hands, their scalps.

Third, a nurturing massage is intense enough to gain your attention but not deep enough to cause you pain. I recommend that you tell the therapist whenever touch is painful. You want to notice and enjoy the experience, not leave more tense because you suffered pain.

I've watched self-esteem grow in client after client. The more touch they receive, the more aware they are of their bodies and, as if by magic, the more self-accepting they become. Healing from low self-esteem comes, not through hiding the body, but by carefully choosing who comes close. If you suffer from low self-esteem, sign up for a massage. You can feel better about yourself with minimal effort. All you have to do is lie there and enjoy!

Celebrate Your Breasts

The important thing is not what they think of me,
it is what I think of them
—QUEEN VICTORIA (1819-1901)

Many of us women feel judged by the size and shape of our breasts. Making peace with our breasts can be central to making peace with ourselves as women. The size and shape of our breasts are often used as a standard for judging our sexual attractiveness. I've worked with women who felt their breasts were too small and some who were embarrassed by how large their breasts were. Women who have lost one or both breasts to cancer may struggle with feeling as if their femininity and appeal were taken along with their mammary tissue.

Take out your body journal and draw a picture of "ideal" breasts and a second picture of your breasts. How are these two pictures similar? How do they differ?

Write out an inner dialogue between you and your breasts, telling them how you feel and letting them respond. If you have had one or both of your breasts removed, write to them the way you would a friend who is no longer in your life. Express your gratitude, your sadness, your pride, and your self-conscious feelings. By communicating with your breasts, you celebrate them and give them the honor due them. Be a queen and let your attitude about yourself matter more than anyone else's opinion of you or any part of your body. Make peace with who you are.

Assess Your Stress

Simplify.
—HENRY DAVID THOREAU (1817-1862)

Too busy? Simplify by saying "no" to new obligations.
Too much clutter around the house? Simplify by having a garage sale.

Too tired? Take the phone off the hook and take a nap.

Too confused to know what to do? Ask your body.

Get out your body journal and draw an outline of your body. Using colored pens or pencils, color in the tense, painful, or tight areas of your body. You may feel a cramp between your shoulder blades, an earache, throbbing in your chest, or lower back pain. Mark in all the areas where you feel discomfort or soreness.

Compare this drawing with the previous ones. Is there a pattern developing? Are some areas of your body chronically affected by stress? Are new areas of your body being affected? If you choose, share your drawings with your body buddy to see if she can shed even more light on what your body is telling you about simplifying your life.

Listen to Your Body

Many people can listen to their cat more intelligently than they can listen to their own despised body. Because they attend to their pet in a cherishing way, it returns their love. Their body, however, may have to let out an earth-shattering scream in order to be heard at all.
—MARION WOODMAN, *The Pregnant Virgin* (1995)

Last week Stud, my opinionated male cat, was angry with me for not allowing him to go outside. He sat with his nose pressed against the doorjamb, occasionally looking over at me with seeming disgust. I didn't feel it was safe for him to go out at that hour, so I picked him up to comfort him. He wailed a protest while glaring at me straight in the eye. He seemed to express rage at what he experienced as mistreatment on my part.

Our bodies are similar. When we make decisions that impinge on our physical well-being, our bodies cry out: a backache, a foot cramp, mild indigestion. If we repeatedly ignore our bodies, the volume increases: a bronchial infection, a spastic colon, a slipped disc. A deeply ingrained hostility toward our bodies may result in a deafening wail: a malignancy, a heart attack, a total collapse. One way or the other, our bodies will speak.

While not all illnesses are the direct result of a poor relationship with our bodies, I agree with Arnold Mindell, who wrote in *Working with the Dreaming Body*, "I don't believe that a person actually creates disease, but that his soul is expressing an important message through the disease." What is the message your body is conveying to you right now? Listen to your body with the same compassion you would give a loved one.

Get a Grip on Dieting

If you have formed the habit of checking out every new diet that
comes along, you will find that, mercifully, they all blur together,
leaving you with only one definite piece of information:
French fried potatoes are out.
—JEAN KERR, *Please Don't Eat the Daisies* (1957)

We are bombarded almost daily with contradictory claims about what foods are good for us, what vitamins we can't live without, in contrast to clever ways to lose weight without having to go without the foods we like, and easy-to-use, no-need-to-sweat exercise equipment. Let's get a grip here.

The fact is, your body has its own unique way of metabolizing food, creating stronger muscle tissue, and generating the energy you need. Rather than take someone else's word for it, check out how your body responds to different foods and types of movement. Ask yourself questions such as, "Am I eating when I'm hungry or in response to an emotional need?" and "Do I feel better after a particular exercise or am I pushing myself too hard to meet some-one else's standards?" Pay more attention to your body than to numbers of calories, listen to your muscles more closely than the commands of the instructor on your aerobics video.

Find and follow your body's rhythm. Do what works for you. If you do, I'll bet you spend your dollars more wisely and save on unneeded diet programs, supplements, exercise equipment, and other paraphernalia.

Trust Your Gut

To the rationally minded the mental processes
of the intuitive appear to work backwards.
—FRANCES WICKES

I was in London years ago emerging from the subway when I said to my traveling buddies, "I know something's off-base here. I can feel it in my gut." I hurried us along to our next stop and didn't give that moment much thought until the next day when we spotted a front-page story at the newsstand. A bomb had exploded at that subway station, killing several travelers a short time after we were there! We all looked at each other in horror, chills running down our spines.

Ever just know something to be true but you're unable to prove it to someone else? Ever have your stomach roll into knots when a particular person walked into the room? Or feel the hair on the back of your neck stand up as you sensed something awful was about to happen?

The process of trusting our bodies is often the reverse of traditional reasoning, which collects the evidence, assesses the data, and then draws a conclusion. But sometimes our bodies tell us the conclusion before the data is available. Trust your gut. There's wisdom down inside of you.

Dine Well

One cannot think well, love well, sleep well,
if one has not dined well.
—VIRGINIA WOOLF (1882-1941)

What is dining well to you? Is a scrumptious meal a plate of steamed veggies and a slice of warm homemade bread? How about a tropical fruit salad with fresh kiwi, pineapple, papaya, and a dollop of yogurt? Or maybe for you, dining well is a thick steak, mashed potatoes, and corn on the cob.

There is no one right way to eat that works for everyone. True, there are some general principles about nutrition. The less fat, the more fresh fruits and vegetables, the better. But I've taken these principles and, at times, turned them into rules, using them as weapons to deprive myself of life's healthy pleasures.

So here is your assignment for today. Dine well. Whatever that means to you. Eat well, enjoy every mouthful to its sensuous, delicious, scrumptious potential. And then expect to think, love, and sleep well as well.

Enjoy!

Expect the Unexpected

Life is not orderly. No matter how we try to make life so, right in the middle of it we die, lose a leg, fall in love, drop a jar of applesauce.
—NATALIE GOLDBERG

I suspect that you are an over-achiever. A woman who wasn't committed to bettering herself wouldn't have the self-discipline to read these entries every day. That's both good and bad news, isn't it?

I mean, we're conscientious, hard-working, and wanting something more for ourselves. But along with these wonderful traits comes a secret (or not so secret) desire to control ourselves and everyone else who will let us.

I know I'd love to control the world. I'd make a number of changes, starting with funding research to find something, anything, wrong with broccoli. I'd make it against the law to get up before 9 A.M. (sorry all you morning people, you've been in control far too long). And I'd initiate a global campaign to convince men that sensible shoes are much sexier than high heels.

But alas, I am not in control of the world. Much of the time I'm not even in control of myself. So, I'm learning to let that be okay. I'm not supposed to be in control. I'm laughing a bit more, worrying a bit less, taking a few more naps, and making shorter to-do lists. Rather than let it all take me by surprise, I'm learning to expect the unexpected. I'm feeling a lot more sane.

Sing with the Children

*Take a music-bath once or twice a week for a few seasons, and you
will find that it is to the soul what the water-bath is to the body.*
—OLIVER WENDELL HOLMES

Lately I've gotten out of the habit of watching the nightly news
and then trying to fall asleep with the sad, violent, and
disconcerting images still dancing in my mind. Instead, I've been
listening to tapes that are soothing and affirming. One tape I
especially enjoy is of a children's choir singing songs full of hope
and encouragement. Since there's no one around to critique my
singing voice, I often join in and sing along with the other kids.

Celebrate your voice by singing with the same enthusiasm you
once did when you were a child. Sing as you did before you knew
you were supposed to sing a particular way or that others might in
any way be critical. Let yourself enjoy being a kid again!

Color outside the Lines

Nobody objects to a woman being a good writer or sculptor or geneticist if at the same time she manages to be a good wife, good mother, good-looking, good-tempered, well-groomed, and unassertive.
—LESLIE M. McINTYRE

Do you color inside the lines? Many of us feel safer following the rules. The reason for this is no mystery. When we were children and broke the rules set down by adults, we were usually punished—a frightening experience. As adults, we naturally feel more at ease when we're cooperating with the ones in power—the boss, the police officer, the doctor—than we are if going against their authority.

Following a strict diet set out for you by someone else can give a sense of safety that may or may not be warranted. Once on a diet, life becomes much simpler, with fewer decisions to make. No longer do you have to think about what to eat or not eat. You can simply follow the diet's rules and your anxiety subsides. The struggle becomes whether or not to follow the rules of the diet.

Even though following a diet may have the illusion of being more responsible, the underlying reality is that you have placed your choices in the hands of someone else. True freedom, along with exercising genuine self-responsibility, will come to you once you create for yourself the eating patterns that reflect your own body's needs and rhythms.

When you draw your own boundaries, you will naturally color outside the lines other people give you. Make your own choices.

Gently Develop Your Sexuality

The process by which we become sexual seems to be less a natural
unfolding of biological tendencies than a social learning process
through which we come to affirm certain sexual meanings in our
interaction with significant others.
—JAMES NELSON, *Embodiment* (1978)

Ideally, we are introduced to sexuality slowly, gently, in step with our age and biological development. But sadly, too few women in this society are graced with that experience. Some experts believe that as many as one-half of the little girls in America are sexually molested. As Roland Summitt, M.D., a child psychiatrist, says, "The one thing a child learns from sexual abuse is how to be abused."

Women who have not been abused may have suffered from a neglected sexuality. Perhaps no one in our growing-up years contributed any affirmation or modeling of healthy sexuality. Not knowing how to be sexual, some of us wonder what appropriate sexuality is.

How would you describe the process by which you became sexual? Were you introduced to sex in age-appropriate stages? Overwhelmed with too much too soon? Or left out in the cold? If any of these things occurred, you may experience issues around sexuality which stem from ignored or disrupted sexual development. Give yourself permission to attend to these wounded and neglected areas.

You may want to talk with a therapist specially trained to help women recover from childhood sexual abuse or neglect. Most communities have support groups of women dealing with these issues as well. You may find a safe haven with women who have similar experiences to your own. Give yourself the opportunity to reclaim your sexuality as your own.

Honor Your Inheritance

We inherit from our ancestors gifts so often taken for granted—our names, the color of our eyes and the texture of our hair, the unfolding of varied abilities and interest in different subjects. . . . Each of us contains within our fragile vessels of skin and bones and cells this inheritance of soul. We are links between the ages, containing past and present expectations, sacred memories and future promise. Only when we recognize that we are heirs can we truly be pioneers.
—Edward C. Sellnor, *Mentoring* (1990)

My legs were inherited from my mother, and the shape of my head came from my father. No one knows where my green eyes came from, since my father's eyes are blue and my mother's are brown. Certainly there were some green-eyed ancestors on both sides back in history somewhere.

Along with these physical attributes, I've also inherited drippy sinuses from my mother's side of the family and migraine headaches from my father's side. Fortunately, both sides of the family have a long life expectancy, usually living well into their eighties and mid-nineties. Altogether, I come from rugged, strong-willed immigrants from Switzerland, Wales, and England.

What have you inherited from your ancestors? Knowing about the health problems and strengths of your family can help you take better care of your body through preventive measures. Record in your body journal the vulnerable areas that may require your attention. And celebrate the strengths that have been passed down to you from your family. Your body is a unique creation, your biological inheritance.

Make Peace with Pain

My body, however, would not let me get away with neglectful
treatment of it and had communicated an important lesson to me:
Our body symptoms have meaning beyond the immediate health
problem they are warning us about.
—CHRISTIANE NORTHRUP, M.D., *Women's Bodies,*
Women's Wisdom (1994)

While I grew up believing that pain was my enemy, I'm
learning a different view of physical suffering, thanks to the
courage of some women I know. A number of my clients have had
serious car accidents, some leaving permanent scars and disabilities
that require coping with pain on a daily basis. With prolonged
pain, it's easy to feel antagonistic towards one's body, since it seems
no matter what is done, nothing eases the agony. At times, separating
from the pain seems the only answer to getting even the simplest of
tasks completed. Otherwise, pain would absorb all one's energy.

What these brave women are teaching me, however, is that
numbing out to reality is a short-term, insufficient solution at best.
Women who are the most successful at regaining a sense of mastery
and satisfaction in their lives are those who look beyond the pain
sensation, diligently searching for what meaning lies beneath the
pain. They've uncovered rage, sadness, disappointment, a fear of
happiness, ambivalence about sex. As each of these jewels is
unearthed and examined, a new level of vitality and passion vibrates
through their lives.

No one asks for pain in order to grow. But when we wrestle with
the pain, rather than ignore or dismiss it, healing results. I stand in
awe of these women who bravely learn pain's lessons rather than
collapse in self-pity and despair.

Take a Bite of Fall

Autumn is the bite of a harvest apple.
—CHRISTINA PETROWSKY

I love the fall. Even though I loved summer as a child, excitement surged through me at the prospect of getting back to school, seeing my friends again after the long vacation, getting new school clothes, and picking out my notebooks. Autumn means different things to different people.

What sensations, aromas, sights, sounds, or tastes remind you of the delights of fall? Take time today to enjoy at least one of these reminders. Join me in honoring fall by sharing a taste that calls to mind the cooling of the air and the leaves changing colors. Bring your body with you into a celebration of the fall by crunching into a fresh harvest apple. Yummy!

Admire Your Body

He that has a great nose thinks everybody is speaking of it.
—THOMAS FULLER

For a Christmas present one year, a man I was dating gave me framed photos of myself that he had taken when we had gone on a picnic together. The photos showed me relaxing in jeans and a tank top. He was proud of himself. I was horrified.

I showed the pictures to a girlfriend of mine and said, "Yuck, look at me! I'm so skinny!"

She stared back at me in surprise, "You look great in these pictures—slim, long, lean. I'd love to look like this."

Then it was my turn to be surprised. I'd long envied her curvaceous body, wishing mine showed some of the same round firmness.

What a waste of time, wishing we had someone else's body. Especially when they may be wishing they looked like us! Take a look at yourself from someone else's eyes and see just how beautiful you are. And enjoy!

Celebrate Your Nose

You have to sniff out joy, keep your nose to the joy-trail.
—Buffy Sainte-Marie, in *Ms. magazine*, 1975

One of my clients told me last week, "Hmmm. . . . I love the smell of your place."

"My place smells?" I asked.

"Yes, it smells like massage oil," she smiled. "I have some clothing with that oil on it and every time I get a whiff of it, I think of being here, nurtured and safe. Coming through the door and catching the scent relaxes me."

Aromas are powerful triggers for memories and emotions. Follow your nose to discover sources of pleasure.

Breathe in the aroma of a sprig of jasmine.

Delight in the body scent of your mate.

Savor the warm fragrance of newly baked bread.

Immerse yourself in the salty scent of a sea breeze or the brisk air of early morning.

Do your nose a favor and sniff out a fragrant joy today.

Breathe Out Blame

Although the world is full of suffering,
it is full also of the overcoming of it.
—HELEN KELLER, *Optimism* (1903)

If you've been hurt by someone else, don't waste time blaming yourself. Instead remind yourself that:

You are not to blame if your house is robbed, even if you left a back window open or forgot to set the burglar alarm. The only person responsible for the theft is the thief.

You are not to blame if your spouse hit you in the face, even if you yelled or said something that upset your partner. The only person responsible for the hitting is the hitter.

You are not to blame for being raped, no matter what you were wearing, where you were walking, or how late it may have been. The only person responsible for the rape is the rapist.

You are not to blame for being molested as a child, even if you didn't tell anyone for years or even if it occasionally felt good. The only person responsible for the molestation is the molester.

This list can go on and on. No matter what you did or didn't do, said or didn't say, wore or didn't wear, tried or didn't try, you are not to blame for the abuse or deprivation you have endured. The only person responsible for the abuse is the abuser.

So, take a deep breath and exhale the blame. Let it go.

Have Faith

Whenever I start dating someone new I ask myself if this is the kind
of man I want my children to spend their weekends with.
—RITA RUDNER, Comedian

Through books, audiocassettes, videotapes, TV, and the Internet, we have access to more information about successful relationships than at any other point in history. And yet divorce is commonplace. Marriages lasting more than seven years are now considered long-term, when a few decades ago marital unions were expected to last a lifetime. It's easy to become cynical about love and romance.

Whether you are currently in a relationship or in-between relationships, let your body help you renew your faith in your ability to be romantically successful. Your body knows when someone is untrustworthy and will tell you through the tightness in your jaw or the pain in your belly. Be cautious of someone who is critical of your body, since sexual intimacy blossoms when your body feels safe. Nothing droops quicker than a libido that's frightened or criticized. You and your body long to be loved, so make sure you bring your body into your romantic relationships.

Whether dealing with a current relationship or a new romance, let your body guide you as you negotiate new terms in your relationship. Ask yourself: Do I feel relaxed and safe with this person? Do I feel desirable? Let your body answer.

Take Charge of Your Health Care

We have been taught the myth about medical gods—that doctors
know more than we do about our bodies, that the experts hold the
cure. It's no wonder that when I ask women to tell me what's going
on in their bodies, they sometimes reply,
"You tell me—you're the doctor!"
—CHRISTIANE NORTHRUP, M.D., *Women's Bodies,*
Women's Wisdom (1994)

A couple of years ago I found a lump in my breast, which a surgeon was anxious to remove. Previously I'd had a fluid-filled cyst that was easily, painlessly drained. The surgeon was unwilling to drain the second lump. Instead, he urged me to plan for surgery within the week.

Shaken, I drove home praying for guidance. By the time I got home, I knew what to do—talk to another doctor about possibly trying to drain the lump, with surgery as a last resort. The next day I called my gynecologist, who was reluctant to contradict the recommendation of the surgeon. But after I insisted, he agreed to try to drain the lump. After he successfully drained it, he sat down across from me, looked me in the eye, and said, "We did it and saved you from surgery. I wouldn't have done this if you hadn't been assertive. You've taken good care of yourself."

I believe that God and my body led me, prompting me to take charge of my own health care and not blindly following the recommendation of one doctor. Any reputable physician will welcome a second, even a third, opinion. If you receive any resistance, find a new doctor. A doctor that isolates you is potentially dangerous to your health. Put your body in charge of your health care. Your body knows the way back to health.

Survey Your Spiritual Journey

The strongest, surest way to the soul is through the flesh.
—MABLE DODGE, *Lorenzo in Taos* (1932)

Write in the numbers indicating how often, if ever, the statements are true. Modify those statements that don't apply to you. 1—Never, 2—Sometimes, 3—Always.

___I am grateful to God for the miracle of my body.

___I feel there is "enough" for me (enough time, love, health, etc.).

___I recognize when my body is degraded through spiritual abuse.

___I regularly reject religious teaching that degrades the body.

___I feel safe in my religious/spiritual community.

___I believe my body is created in God's image.

___I believe that God loves my body, all of my body.

___I draw spiritual strength through grounding my body.

___I explore new ways to include my body in my spiritual journey.

___If I fast, I do so in a healthy way.

___I pray daily, letting go of what I cannot control.

___I feel I am doing what I was meant to do with my life.

___I rarely, if ever, feel all alone.

___I learn more about God the more I learn about my body.

___I regularly receive massage to enhance my spiritual life.

Scoring Evaluation

37-45 Congratulations! You enjoy an embodied spirituality.

26-36 Watch out. Your spirituality is at odds with your body.

0-25 Body alert! Your body is endangered by your spirituality.

Don't Be Fooled

Advertisers do not want us to feel good about our body.
If we did, we might not feel a need to buy their wares.
—CARL KOCH AND JOYCE HEIL, *Created in God's Image* (1991)

Here's an eye-opening exercise you can do alone or with your body buddy. Program your VCR to tape four hours of TV, any commercial channel, any time of day. Then play back the tape, only, instead of skipping the commercials, skip the programs. Record in your body journal how many commercials base their ads on there being something wrong, inadequate, or unacceptable about your body. Also notice how many products, even if they do not directly address a body concern (like cars, telephones, or other gadgets and appliances), use bodies or subliminal promises of sex as a lure. Then write down all the negative body statements made in the ads. See how many of these messages you and your body buddy can find.

Your findings may amaze you! We are barraged by little sound bites nipping away at our sense of satisfaction with our bodies. This distorted information is designed to sell products, not make your or my life better. We cannot and must not allow these ads to undermine our relationships with our bodies. The key is to be aware of these subtle and blatant messages. As we get better at recognizing them, we can sooner reject them.

Once you've made your list, cut them into one "untruism" per piece of paper. With your body buddy, rip each of the items up, while reciting the truth about your body. For example, the message, "I am too old and unattractive to be loved" can be obliterated while proclaiming, "I am lovable at any age." Keep going until all the messages are destroyed. Welcome to your freedom.

Act on a New Assumption

The first problem for all of us, men and women, is not to learn,
but to unlearn, to clear out some of the old assumptions.
—GLORIA STEINEM, "A New Egalitarian Life Style,"
The New York Times (August 26, 1971)

Prior to my first body work session, I assumed that my body was a possession and that my job was to discipline it into submission, so that it would take me wherever I needed to go. I acted on this assumption for over thirty years, until I ended up in bed, utterly overcome with exhaustion, depression, and a sense of failure.

Fortunately, I've had the opportunity to discard this false assumption and develop a more life-enhancing way to look at myself. My body and I are one and the same, valuable, wise, and worthy of care. Instead of telling my body what to do, now I listen.

Identify one negative assumption you have about your body. Write it out so that you can see it clearly. Then list the destructive outcomes that acting on this assumption has had on your health, your relationships, and your outlook. Now write out an assumption you want to adopt in its stead. Take time to act on this new assumption today.

Celebrate Taste

Sour, sweet, bitter, pungent, all must be tasted.
—CHINESE PROVERB

So often we fall into a rut, eating the same foods, sometimes hardly tasting the bites as they go down.

Today, treat yourself to a tasting feast. Seek out a type of cooking you don't ordinarily eat and order something a little bit daring. Sample something spicy, munch on a new type of soft and chewy bread, sip an exotic blend of tea, and try a wickedly saucy dessert. Celebrate all the areas on your tongue!

Say "Ouch" When It Hurts

For us to experience pleasure,
we must also be willing to risk experiencing pain.
—CAROL C. WELL, *Right-Brain Sex* (1989)

Some clients find it surprising that I request they tell me if there is pain during a massage. They assume that the more pain they can tolerate the better.

I believe that pain is the body's way of telling us that we are being damaged and that we should stop what we are doing. The goal of my body work is to help people release stress in a comfortable way and to increase their ability to experience pleasure. That requires that they risk experiencing pain. It does not mean that they must experience pain.

I used to think pain was a requirement for me to be close to someone else. Because of this distorted notion, I tolerated abuse from others and minimized the damage I was suffering. After years of hurt, I've come to see that the pleasure of healthy intimacy comes with the possibility of pain, not the necessity, obligation, or acceptability of pain.

Follow your body's lead. Say "ouch" when it hurts and demand that changes be made, whether the pain be physical or emotional. Listen to the pain. It is there to guide you.

Tell the Truth

She who conceals her disease cannot expect to be cured.
—ETHIOPIAN PROVERB

One of the secret shames among women is the eating disorder, bulimia, which is characterized by binge eating and then purging activities. Purging may include vomiting, laxative abuse, fasting, or rigid dieting. A bulimia sufferer may be overweight, underweight, or of average weight.

Barbara McFarland and Rodney Susong, in *Killing Ourselves with Kindness*, list the major symptoms of bulimia as binge eating, depressed moods and self-deprecating thoughts, extreme feelings of guilt after a binge, preoccupation with food and weight, fear of losing control once a binge has begun, a deep sense of inadequacy and helplessness, and feeling isolated. Perhaps the most seriously dangerous part of this disease is the desire in the woman struggling with bulimia to hide her pain from view.

Whether we suffer from an eating disorder or not, we all are hiding some wound, hurt, or failing from those around us. Take courage today and call one woman you trust or you know loves you. Just one. And tell her the truth about your pain. Let her join you; let her help you take another step toward coming home to your body.

Refresh Yourself with Water

Two-thirds of your body is composed of water, making it your body's
most vital nutrient. Water provides a valuable source of minerals,
like calcium and magnesium. Helps digest food and absorb nutrients
into the body. Carries nutrients to organs via the bloodstream.
—DON R. POWELL, *365 Health Hints* (1990)

The late afternoon doldrums are common for many of us. Our bodies need a rest from the work routine. But instead, most of us force ourselves to work through without a break. We guzzle a cup or two of coffee and blearily push on. Today, instead of drinking coffee, try drinking several large glasses of water. You may be surprised at how refreshing water can be.

Not only will drinking water help to revive you, you'll feel full and less likely to snack on unwanted cookies or coffee. Plus, this afternoon water treat will help you reach your daily goal of eight glasses. For a special treat, garnish the water with lemon, strawberries, or lime slices. Make it fun!

Be Positive, Be Realistic

We have been taught to believe that negative equals realistic
and positive equals unrealistic.
—SUSAN JEFFERS

In my workshops I ask participants to list the things they don't feel they have enough of. Without hesitation, the group members offer up things like money, time, energy, support, friends, leisure, sex. Living out of a feeling of scarcity is a way of life for many of us. When we feel we don't have enough, we often feel like we are not good enough or not doing enough, and push our bodies to perform.

Affirming possibilities, recognizing opportunities, and declaring ourselves acceptable are not activities that flow from a perspective of scarcity. We must believe in abundance, in goodness, in love for these life-affirming attitudes to arise.

Is your view of reality based on a sense of deprivation, inadequacy, and scarcity? Or are you asserting a perspective of abundance? Our views of abundance or scarcity are rooted in our view of God. Do you see God as adequate or inadequate? Attentive or absent? Nurturing or abusive?

Only when we believe that God is adequate can we experience ourselves as sufficient for the task of living. Only when we feel that there is enough for us can we accept that we are enough and stop running.

Look underneath Your Craving

I know well what I am fleeing from
but not what I am in search of.
—MICHEL DE MONTAIGNE (1533-1592)

One of my clients described how the previous night she had eaten a dozen doughnuts, a bag of potato chips, and a box of Oreos. "I had such a craving to eat," she said sadly. "For a while I felt calmer, but then guilt and self-hatred hit me like a tidal wave. I feel so needy, but I can't figure out what it is I really need."

I know how she feels. Sometimes a desire beyond words propels me to try anything to stop the longing. The question to ask ourselves, however, is not how to stop the craving, but, "What lies underneath the craving?" My client didn't really need doughnuts, potato chips, or Oreos. Something more profound, more important lay beneath her sense of neediness. Perhaps she was feeling anger that she had been taught to suppress. Maybe a need for affection had been ignored since childhood. Perhaps her craving covered her fear to take a career risk and actually go for what she had secretly wanted to do but hadn't told a soul.

Underneath a craving that aims us at self-destructive behavior is usually a legitimate need that deserves our attention. Don't wait until you are so needy that "now" feels too late. Ask yourself, "What is underneath my craving?" Then check in with your body and expect an answer through a phrase that may go through your mind, a picture, a memory, or some other form of insight.

Locate Fear in Your Body

*To fear is one thing. To let fear grab you by the tail
and swing you around is another.*
—KATHERINE PATERSON, *Jacob Have I Loved* (1980)

Fear grabs my body in the gut, like a fist squeezing my stomach in an iron grip. My legs pull up, my spine curves, and eating is the last thing on earth I want to do. I may not always feel frightened, but I know that if I've lost my appetite, there's something going on that scares me. Paying attention to my body alerts me to ask myself, "What is frightening me now?"

How does your body carry fear? Your body may have the opposite reaction to mine, with a longing to binge on comfort food. Your head may ache, your teeth may chatter, or your feet may feel ticklish. Notice how your body communicates fear, and record this information in your body journal. As you and your body work together, you'll be more able to identify dangerous situations or relationships and more adept at protecting yourself from harm.

Celebrate Your Bones

Though most women start to think of bone loss only at menopause, it often begins years before. In fact, up to 50 percent of the bone that women lose over their lifespan is lost before menopause even begins.
—CHRISTIANE NORTHRUP M.D., *Women's Bodies, Women's Wisdom* (1994)

Are you giving your bones the attention they need to stay strong and sturdy throughout your life?

Women are especially vulnerable to bone deterioration as we age. Even though our bodies contain more calcium, which is required for healthy bones, than any other mineral, our bodies do not manufacture this needed substance. We have to get all the calcium we need from diet alone. According to the Food and Nutrition Board of the National Academy of Sciences, teenagers need 1,200 milligrams of calcium a day, and those of us over eighteen need 800 milligrams a day. Other experts claim that if a woman is over forty, she needs 1,500 milligrams of calcium a day.

Let your bones know you care by eating foods high in calcium and, as your doctor recommends, a mineral supplement. Dairy products, salmon, tofu, and almonds can help give your bones the calcium they need. Be good to your bones; they deserve your attention.

Risk

Risk! Risk anything! Care no more for the opinions of others,
for those voices. Do the hardest thing on earth for you.
Act for yourself. Face the truth.
—KATHERINE MANSFIELD, *The Journal of Katherine Mansfield* (1927)

I went to the Humane Society to find a companion for my cat, Sassy. There, curled up in the corner of a cage, was a little black furball with white whiskers who would soon come home with me and answer to the name Stud. He was quite safe in his cage at the Humane Society, protected from other larger animals, cars, and disease that might have otherwise threatened him. But he was also unhappy alone there in his risk-free cage. He faced no challenges. He lay in the corner with his head resting on his paws, awake and yet disinterested in his world.

Like Stud, we all need challenges to be happy and healthy. While it is foolish to take unnecessary risks, it is equally foolish to hide from challenges. Sometimes the most dangerous thing we can do is play it safe. It can be dangerous allowing advertisers to shape your self-image. It can be dangerous to blindly follow a doctor's advice without being clear about your options or asking for a second (or third or fourth) opinion. It can be dangerous allowing friends or family members to criticize your body, creating a sense of dis-ease inside of you. Sometimes the safest path in the long run appears to be the most challenging in the short run. Safety can become a cage in which your spirit and body shrivel and die. Make the risky choice, take on the challenge, and wrestle with your personal experience of the truth.

NOVEMBER

COCOON

She felt her skin—
once microscopic layers—
grow thick and dense;
her body, rubber-like,
lose sensation;
tongue and lips
harden
around a silenced sentence;
brain cells
tingle with induced sleep.
It was a matter now
of holding on,
of trying to endure
this great death
without giving in
to the temptation
to hasten it.
It happened so naturally;
this cocoon
of numbed forgetfulness
steadily wrapped itself
around and through her.
She could only hope
to find a way to breathe
and wait for spring.

Increase Your Enjoyment Comfort Zone

Everybody needs more love. More love. More love. More love. The truth is that nobody had a perfect childhood and none of us got enough praise, attention, recognition, affection, coddling, cuddling, blessing, or encouragement. We all need more love now.
—DAPHNE ROSE KINGMA, *True Love* (1991)

Most of us have what I call an enjoyment comfort zone, an invisible line we draw around ourselves that allows in pleasure, nurturance, and love while protecting us from hurtful experiences. The problem with making this wall too solid is that we may keep out the positive experiences we and our bodies desperately need.

Today's project is to move that line a little further out. Don't try to tear down the wall; you still need it for protection against harmful people and possibilities. But you'll be safe if you push it out just a little bit further and let a tiny bit more pleasure in.

How? Try one new thing today that makes room for more love for your body. Listen for that compliment on your appearance and embrace it by saying "Thank you," rather than rejecting it with an "Oh, it's nothing." Let your mate know that you'd like some cuddling time and a foot rub when you get home tonight. If you're especially daring, call up a good friend and say, "I've been discouraged. Would you tell me one thing you like about my body?"

We all need love. Disembodied love is no love at all. Whatever you do today to enlarge your enjoyment comfort zone, be mindful of your body. Open yourself to more embodied love.

Squeeze Stress Out Your Toes

Whether it be a sip of wine, a shopping spree, a well-deserved vacation, a vigorous laugh, or a satisfying cry—such small indulgences can brighten and enliven our lives.
—ROBERT ORNSTEIN AND DAVID SOBEL, *Healthy Pleasures* (1989)

A girlfriend of mine told me about a small indulgence she enjoys at the end of every day. Right before she falls off to sleep, she stretches her body, squeezing the tension down her body and out her toes. Starting at her scalp, she gently stretches her face, neck, shoulders, arms, torso, and legs until she envisions squeezing the day's stress down to her feet, like she might press toothpaste out of its tube. Finally, she stretches her toes, milking the tension completely out of her body. Fully relaxed, she easily falls asleep.

Tonight, help yourself fall asleep by letting go of the day's stress. Squeeze the tension down your body and out your toes. Sleep well.

Don't "Should" on Yourself

Between two evils, I always pick the one I never tried before.
—MAE WEST, *Klondike Annie* (1936)

Ever get caught up in all the "shoulds" of life?
I do. First, there are all the shoulds I get from others. I should be a helpful, kind person. I should nurture my friends. I should contribute to worthy causes. I should never let anyone down. I should always be on time. . . .

And now that I'm learning how to care for my body, I have a whole new list of shoulds. I should eat better. I should exercise more. I should get massages more often. I should smell the roses and appreciate my nose. I should pay attention to my breath. I should listen to all my illnesses so that I can learn from my body.

Whew!

Today, let all of the shoulds go. Treat yourself to something just a little bit wicked, like a juicy, fat-filled cheeseburger, fries, and a chocolate shake, or maybe a huge slice of cheesecake with cherries on top. I think I'm going for deep-fried taquitos smothered in guacamole, with refried beans with melted cheese on the side. Some days we just have to embrace our shadow side if we're going to survive being so wonderful!

Be Content with What You Have

Until you make peace with who you are,
you'll never be content with what you have.
—DORIS MORTMAN

Remember the adage, "When the going gets tough, the tough go shopping"? Women carry the stigma of being avid shoppers, if not addicted to spending money as a means of managing their emotions. I've certainly found shopping for a new outfit or purchasing new items for my home to be a way of bolstering my drooping self-esteem or giving me extra encouragement after a disappointment.

But putting a gorgeous outfit over a body I hate will not make me feel good about myself. In fact, nothing I can buy or could ever own will satisfy my deepest longings. Contentment is possible only through resolving my negative feelings regarding my body. Rather than spending an afternoon shopping, my time would be better spent getting a massage, having an inner dialogue with my body, or attending a body-oriented support group. Putting effort into dealing with the problem directly is never a waste of time (or money).

If you want to be content with what you have, then be content with who you are. When we are at peace with our bodies, we can enjoy what we wear and what we own, because we no longer expect these objects to emotionally heal us. Objects can't nurture us. Only love can heal.

Locate Confusion in Your Body

*It is while trying to get everything straight in my head
that I get confused.*
—MARY VIRGINIA MICKA, *Oddly Enough* (1990)

Confusion can spin us around, sending us running off in directions we never planned. Rather than allow your quandaries to get the best of you, let your body help you regain your bearings and decide what step to take.

Start by locating confusion in your body. A tightness in your forehead as your eyes squint, perplexed? A rigid spine as you twirl in the fog? Toes curled upward, pulling your feet off the ground? What is the unique way your body lets you know you're befuddled and bewildered? To regain a sense of clarity, try standing equally on both legs, allowing your arms to hang comfortably and take several deep breaths. You'll be more able to think clearly when you are calm. And don't forget, in all the confusion, to record this information in your body journal. Once things are sorted out, you'll need what you learned in this process. Share your confusion with someone who can help bring clarity to your situation.

Celebrate Smell

Who knows? Our nose.
—CARL KOCH AND JOYCE HEIL, *Created in God's Image* (1991)

I could smell something burning, something odd, a scent of danger. "Oh, I left something cooking on the stove!" I shouted and ran downstairs to find pasta dark and smoldering on the bottom of the pan. Thanks to my nose, I was alerted before anything burst into flames.

How has your nose helped you to avoid trouble? Did your nose ever alert you to gas fumes from a leaking pipe? Have you detected that someone you feared was approaching when you smelled familiar perfume? Has the stale scent of cigarette smoke alerted you to the health hazards of second-hand smoke? Celebrate your sense of smell today by writing in your body journal how your nose has protected you from danger.

Assess Your Stress

*[I]f we overload ourselves with stress in an unrelenting effort
towards more and more achievements, we can literally die trying,
and quite prematurely at that.*
—DEANE JUHAN, *Job's Body* (1987)

Balance, balance, balance. Ever get tired of hearing about balancing the myriad aspects of our lives? I do. Sometimes learning more about stress management stresses me out.

It would be simpler if someone could tell us specifically what to do to create balance. But no one but you knows for sure how balance is best achieved in your life. You may function at your optimal level with six hours of sleep, love an early morning workout, and feel refreshed by others' company. Or you might need nine hours of sleep, feel healthiest with an afternoon workout, and relax through solitude. Only you, with your body's help, know what you need.

To make things even more challenging, your balance point, which is different from mine, may change from day to day. When your stress level is low, your need for sleep may be less, with more energy for exercise. However, during more demanding times, more sleep may be required for you to maintain your emotional and physical equilibrium. Some days' stress may require an afternoon nap.

Draw a picture of your body in your body journal and color in the tense places. Write a short description about how balance is best created today. Maintaining balance in our lives is not a stagnant endeavor, but requires tuning into our bodies on a daily, if not a moment by moment basis. By being aware of increasing or decreasing stress in our neck muscles, the calm or unrest in our stomachs, or the cramping or relaxing of our pelvic muscles, we can continually assess what is needed to keep our balance.

Learn Leisurely

There can be no education without leisure, and without leisure,
education is worthless.
—SARAH JOSEPHA HALE, *Godey's Lady's Book* (circa 1837)

My memories of school are full of frantically studying for exams, writing papers until the sun came up, and anxiously awaiting the posting of grades. No wonder it seems I've forgotten more than I learned.

When we're anxious, our cognitive abilities are impaired. We learn best in a safe, supportive atmosphere with ample time to digest and discuss new information. So, take some time to rest. Make no conscious effort to learn anything new or produce any grand insight. Simply relax and open yourself up to whatever your body wants to teach you.

Follow Your Inner Clock

People are beginning to resist the rhythm of the machine and suspect
that the path of inner harmony and health
demands an inward attention.
—GAY GAER LUCE, "Trust Your Body Rhythms,"
Psychology Today (April, 1975)

In an astonishing study of newborns, researchers discovered that if parents imposed a sleep and feeding schedule regulated by the clock, their babies had difficulty sleeping at night. However, if parents followed the babies' natural sleep patterns, allowing them to sleep when they were tired and eat when they were hungry, by the second week of life their bodies acclimated to being awake during the day and asleep at night. In one week!

Many parents wrestle with their children over sleeping and eating. Many of our own parents were influenced by parenting practices that forced rigid time frames onto our early biological functions, such as a feeding every four hours even if we were hungry earlier, followed by a nap whether we were sleepy or not. Too few of our parents trusted the wisdom of our little bodies. They believed that their job was to make our bodies conform to their time schedule. At that very early age many of us were taught a terrible lesson—to ignore the rhythm of our bodies and conform to the clock.

Are you still mistreating your body by ignoring the wisdom of your biological rhythms? Imagine how your daily schedule would change if you slept when you were tired and ate when you were hungry. Would you go to bed earlier? Later? Eat fewer meals? More meals? Don't let the artificial time slots created to organize society control the choices you make about your life. Your body is much wiser than the timepiece ticking on your wall.

Deal with Death

I . . . began to recognize that death and destruction were part of the creative process and to see that my body was part of the larger rhythm of endings and beginnings.
—MARJORY ZOET BANKSON, *This is My Body:*
Creativity, Clay, and Change (1993)

None of us can become more connected to our bodies without also becoming more aware of the cycle of birth, death, and resurrection. Birth and rebirth are inspiring, even fun, to talk about. But the death part—well, I'd rather ignore it.

Perhaps our desire to turn our heads away from death is, in part, what motivates us to turn away from our own bodies. No matter how well we care for our bodies, at some point in the future, we will die. Our bodies remind us of our inevitable death in small ways every day—the new lines that form around our eyes, the wisps of gray in our hair, the need to pick off the peppers from the pizza because they now give us heartburn.

Making peace with our bodies brings us face to face with the challenge of making peace with death. This is perhaps one of the most significant and difficult challenges of our lives. Take some time today and contemplate your view of death. Does it frighten you? If so, in what way? Do you have old business to attend to? Is it time to start? Perhaps talk with a trusted friend and come to terms, a little bit more, with an experience that you will, at some point, face.

Celebrate Your Chest

*Pleasing yourself with special treats from time to time
is vital to a healthy, satisfying life.*
—ROBERT ORNSTEIIN AND DAVID SOBEL, *Healthy Pleasures* (1989)

Treat yourself to an energizing self-massage that will lift your shoulders and your outlook on life. Many of us whose shoulders sag need to stretch the muscles on the front of our chests, muscles that might have contracted and even shrunk due to chronically poor posture. Not only do we look a bit bedraggled in this position, but our sad-looking posture can trigger sad feelings inside of us, even when there's nothing external to feel sad about.

Celebrate your chest by sitting up straight in a comfortable chair, feet relaxed on the floor. Take a deep breath and exhale. On the second inhale, slowly extend your arms to either side as if ready to catch a giant beach ball. Bring your arms together on the exhale.

Next tap your upper chest area with the tips of your fingers. Work from your collar bone to the tops of your breasts and then between your breasts. Vary the strength of the tapping, first lighter then deeper, making sure you avoid bruising yourself. Breathe deeply as you tap, allowing the tension you hold in your chest to melt away.

Heal a Childhood Wound

In extreme youth, in our most humiliating sorrow, we think we are alone. When we are older we find that others have suffered too.
—SUSANNE MOARNY

Remember that time when you were a little girl and the kids made fun of you? Maybe you were teased for wearing glasses, being chubby, for having ears that stuck out, or lots of freckles. I don't know which one of your particular physical traits was singled out for ridicule, but I've rarely talked with any woman who wasn't made to feel badly about her body in some way when she was a girl.

When we are children, our sense of humiliation isolates us. Indeed, isolation is the very thing our peers try to achieve, making themselves feel like they belong at our expense. But now, as women, we can use that same experience of abuse to gather together and draw close to one another.

Talk with other women today about experiences they've had in which their bodies were ridiculed or criticized. It will be painful, perhaps, dredging those memories up. But soon you'll find a camaraderie, and maybe even some comedy, in the situation. Allow yourselves to bemoan, grieve, and even laugh together about those girlhood woes, and heal each other in the present.

Celebrate Your Tongue

I was dumb and silent,
I refrained even from good;
And my sorrow grew worse.
My heart was hot within me;
While I was musing the fire burned;
Then I spoke with my tongue.
—PSALM 39:2,3, *New American Standard Bible*

One of the most versatile and useful muscles in our body is our tongue. We can taste, spit, kiss, whistle, swallow, and lick with our tongues. Perhaps most important, we can speak.

Women who do not speak openly about their feelings, their past experiences, and their pain often express their reality in unconscious or self-damaging ways. But when we use our tongues to tell the truth about what we've seen, heard, felt, tasted, and smelled, our bodies can relax into positions of ease and health. Our eyes come back into focus, our heads rise up, our jaws relax, our breathing deepens, and our feet settle back to earth.

Use your tongue to tell the truth. First, write out something you have wanted to say or needed to share with someone. After you have described your feelings or the situation completely, share this information with your body buddy. If there is someone else with whom you need to confide, share with him or her what you have written in your body journal. Invite your body buddy to join you if you need extra support. Your entire body will thank you.

Extend Your Senses

*I think the one lesson I have learned is
that there is no substitute for paying attention.*
—DIANE SAWYER, Journalist

If you're awake, smoke from even a small fire will warn you of potential danger in your home. But when you are asleep, a fire can be fully blazing before you may be alerted. In some cases, smoke inhalation or poisonous gases released from the fire can inhibit your ability to wake, putting your life and your loved ones in jeopardy. The National Bureau of Standards claims that up to eighty percent of all fire deaths occur in residences. At least half of these could have been prevented with smoke detectors.

Even though I set my detector off, from time to time, with my version of cooking, having functional smoke detectors is a simple, inexpensive way to extend your senses. The detector is set off when it gets a whiff of smoke, sounding a loud alarm. Your nose may not detect the smoke, but your ears will definitely pick up on the blaring noise of the alarm.

Protect your home, your life, and the lives of those you live with by extending your senses. Install smoke detectors in your home and sleep easier.

Ask for Help

*Just being in a room with myself is
almost more stimulation than I can bear.*
—KATE BRAVERMAN, *Lithium for Medea* (1989)

E ver get yourself so worked up you thought your head would explode or your heart would burst? Have you ever imagined you had a disease you heard about, or that you were unexpectedly pregnant (and didn't want to be)? Left to your own imagination, have you scared yourself about some situation, assuming all the worst things that could happen until your pulse was racing and your toes were curled?

Sometimes we need the help of others to calm us down so that we can leave the agitated or flooded states, returning to the alert state where we belong. If you are suffering due to an inability to calm yourself, the solution is simple. Call your body buddy or another woman you trust and ask for help.

Together you can explore ways you can use your body to settle down. Does taking a walk help? Talking it out? Getting a hug? Drinking some tea? Let her help you feel safe enough to relax into the alert state.

Recall Your Memory

I can never remember things I didn't understand in the first place.
—AMY TAN, *The Joy Luck Club* (1989)

Write in the numbers indicating how often, if ever, the statements are true. Modify those statements that don't apply to you. 1—Never, 2—Sometimes, 3—Always.

___I trust my body to give me accurate information about the past.

___I trust myself to decide what is true about my past.

___I pay attention if I feel cut off from my body.

___I pay attention if all or parts of my body feel numb.

___I pay attention if feelings seem to come out of nowhere.

___I pay attention to sounds that remind me of past hurts.

___I pay attention to aromas that remind me of past hurts.

___I pay attention to tastes that remind me of past hurts.

___I pay attention to sensations that remind me of past hurts.

___I pay attention to mental images that remind me of past hurts.

___I appropriately express my feelings over the past.

___I can remember my entire childhood.

___My body helps me stay in the safety of the present.

___I trust God to help me heal from past trauma or neglect.

___I know I have the right to know about my past.

___I regularly receive body work to assist in healing painful memories.

Scoring Evaluation

37-45   Great! You are dealing effectively with your past.

26-36   Watch out. Parts of your past are unresolved.

0-25   Body alert! You need to ask for help in resolving past hurts.

Be in Your Body, Be in the Present

I was regretting the past and fearing the future. Suddenly God was
speaking. "My name is 'I Am,'" I waited. God continued.
"When you live in the past, with its mistakes and regrets, it is hard.
I am not there. My name is not 'I was.'
"When you live in the future, with its problems and fears, it is hard.
I am not there. My name is not 'I will be.'
"When you live in this moment, it is not hard. I am here. My name
is 'I Am.'"
—HELEN MELLICOST, *One Hundred Gates*

God gave us bodies as a reliable way to stay in the present. Our bodies are destined to live only in the now. While our minds can be transported to past events or worry over an uncertain future, our bodies content themselves with being right here, at this moment. Our bodies are connected to the past but can no longer live there. We can prepare our bodies for our future plans, but they cannot exist alongside our imaginations. No matter where we go in our minds, we can rely on our bodies to keep us connected to the present moment, the grounded reality of today.

Have you become agitated by past losses or future fancies? Are you lost in the maze of confusing emotion and information over-load? Follow your body back to the present. Sit quietly in a comfortable chair, with the soles of your feet firmly planted on the ground. Close your eyes and take in a deep, slow breath. Feel the air flow inside you, through you, all the way down to your toes. Feel your feet on the ground. Feel the earth holding you safely. Repeat this process for several minutes until you feel firmly planted on the ground, fully inhabiting your body. Breathe a sigh of relief and thank God for giving you a way to make it back home.

Be Encouraged

I always believed that if you set out to be successful,
then you already are.
—KATHERINE DUNHAM

Every so often I get discouraged. Hard to believe, I know, being the perfect woman that I am. But I must confess that I set goals for myself that I do not always meet. Feeling disappointed in myself, I think, "What's the use, Carmen. You'll never make it."

When those negative voices come into my head, I know I've slipped back into my addiction to perfection. Black-and-white thinking takes over with only rigid results available such as good or bad, right or wrong, success or failure. If I make a mistake, then I'm bad, wrong, and a failure. Period. End of discussion.

When I am in touch with my body's process of continual death and regeneration, it's impossible to think in these false terms. My body is a complicated, marvelous living event in which parts are dying, healing, expanding, shrinking, and changing all the time. Every change is part of the process. I don't breathe once a day, but continually. My fingernails grow, are cut, and continue to grow. Waste products are released through my skin, skin that also takes in moisture from lotions and vitamins from the sun. As I cooperate with the ebb and flow of my body's process, I move out of black-and-white thinking and into choosing life.

Choose life. Let the complexity of your body encourage you to accept the complexities of your own soul and life. Feel the surge of success simply by being a part of this miraculous design.

Protect Your Body Image

Some people give us positive messages about our body; other people
send us negative messages. All these bits of information
help compose our body image, but over forming
this image we do have some control.
—CARL KOCH AND JOYCE HEIL, *Created in God's Image* (1991)

I believe one's self-image develops through relating with others. Essentially, I see myself as I believe you see me. I build my self-image on what I think I see in your eyes.

This process can be problematic since I rely on my perception of others, which may or may not be accurate. For example, if I'm rudely treated by a clerk, I may conclude I'm not as appealing as another customer who gets all the help she needs. The clerk's rudeness may have nothing to do with my acceptability. Perhaps I look like a loved one with whom the clerk has recently argued. Or the clerk may be attracted to me, yet rude out of fear that I'll be rejecting (haven't you ever acted strange with someone you wanted to like you?). Or the clerk may simply be in a foul mood.

Protect yourself (especially your bodyself) from letting negative perceptions from strangers or loved ones lower your self-regard. If you feel someone is disapproving, check it out rather than let this experience put an additional barrier between you and your body. Most of the time, when I've spoken with the "disapproving person" or others involved, I've learned that the conclusions I had drawn were off-base.

And if I find that a person actually does reject me or parts of my body, it may be time to end that relationship, even with those who are close to us. Who needs such abuse?

Celebrate Your Face

When we are troubled or making an effort to concentrate, our
forehead and temples can often become tense and congested.
Indeed, over time many people develop worry lines,
which age them considerably.
—Robert Thé, *5-Minute Massage* (1995)

Even in southern California, the air turns briskly cold this time of year, challenging us to take special care of our skin. Treat yourself to a fruity fall mask.

If you have a working fireplace, light a fire and put on soothing music to set the mood. Warm two tablespoons of apricot oil and two tablespoons of cream in a small pan over a low flame on your stove. While the oil is heating, cut a piece of muslin the size of your face with holes for your mouth, eyes, and nose. Soak the muslin in the warmed moisture, making sure it isn't too hot to touch your skin. Squeeze the excess moisture from the muslin, then, lying in a relaxed position, smooth the muslin over your face (being careful to avoid your eyes) and enjoy the warmth for ten to fifteen minutes. After gently removing the muslin, wipe your face clean and apply your toner. Your skin will be replenished with moisture, calcium, and vitamin A.

Put Yourself First

I'm so angry that my body's all but bursting into flame.
—ALAMANDA (1165-1199) in MEG BODIN,
The Women Troubadours (1976)

I remember my first night in self-defense class. Mark, our padded instructor, showed us how to deliver a strike to the head. When it was my turn, I nervously walked onto the mat.

"Take your elbow," he instructed, "and strike me in the head." I feebly popped his face mask with my elbow.

"Hit me!" he bellowed, "Hit me hard!"

"But I'm afraid I'll hurt you!" I said, dropping my hands to my side.

Many of us are afraid to make any effort to protect ourselves because we fear that in expressing our own rage we will hurt other people. We don't want to be like those who have hurt us. Generally speaking, the ability to empathize allows us, in our own decision-making process, to take into account the impact on all concerned. However, when we are being physically attacked or endangered by another person, anger helps us do what needs to be done, to put our needs for safety first with minimal concern for the abusive person's well-being. Out of a misguided fear of hurting someone else, many of us channel our anger away from rather than toward those who threaten to violate us.

Put your body's safety above the well-being of anyone intent on physically hurting you. Refusing to protect ourselves from someone who threatens us is a distortion of the value we women place on protecting our children and those we love. When someone comes uninvited into your personal space, don't be empathetic—defend yourself.

Reject Blame, Embrace Responsibility

A diet counselor once told me that all overweight people are angry with their mothers and channel their frustrations into overeating. So I guess that means all thin people are happy, calm, and have resolved their Oedipal entanglements.
—WENDY WASSERSTEIN, Playwright

It's quite faddish today for experts to offer simplistic answers to complicated problems. Look at the ads. You're promised quick, easy relief for whatever ails you. Just buy.

Buying simplistic explanations can be quite dangerous because of the hidden blame in quick-fix solutions. If the diet, the wrinkle cream, the therapy, the relationship video, the prayer, the cure-all doesn't work, the hidden message is that you are at fault. If you had more faith, more self-control, a better relationship with your parents, a more stringent exercise program, more of the product line, then everything would be great. Since you don't . . . well, you know how this song goes.

I am learning to be very careful about whose opinion I let shape me, because I've been—in fact, I am—shaped emotionally and physically by those I let myself believe. I'm opening myself to the wisdom of those women and men who demonstrate kindness, patience, and awareness of the complexities of the human condition. And when, not if, things don't go smoothly, there is support, not blame available to me.

Be Thankful for Your Age

Old age transfigures or fossilizes.
—MARIE VON EBNER-ESCHENBACK, *Aphorisms* (1905)

Thanksgiving is a time to reflect on the people, experiences, and things for which we're grateful. Few of us would put "getting older" on our list of things we appreciate. Take a few moments and re-examine how our attitudes about aging impact the length and quality of our lives.

My attitude about being a woman who is growing older stresses me out. Let's face it. We live in a society that worships youth. There's not a big market for wrinkles and sags. And, some experts claim that the body is designed to live over a hundred years, but because we mismanage stress, we age much faster and die much younger. Therefore, my stress about my age may be shortening my life span!

We'll be happier and live longer if we challenge these unrealistic attitudes, beginning with ourselves. What attitudes do you have about aging that undermine your acceptance of your body? Are you disappointed in the way your skin is aging? Is your hair turning gray or changing texture? Do your joints ache a little more, causing you to move more slowly than you did in the past? How can you find new and transforming ways to relate to the changes in your body that aging can bring? How can you embrace the new texture of your skin? Alter the way you style your hair? Try out new ways of stretching and moving to maximize your flexibility? Be thankful for your age and transfigure your losses into pluses.

Calm Yourself to Sleep

Oh sleep! it is a gentle thing,
Beloved from pole to pole!
—SAMUEL TAYLOR COLERIDGE (1772-1834)

When I'm anxious, I can have a terrible time falling asleep. First, I try to calm myself by reading a detective novel. Perhaps I play a few hands of solitaire. I feed Sassy a handful of her favorite kitty snack and rub Stud's tummy until he purrs. The light goes off. Then the light goes back on and I check out one more chapter, play another quick hand of solitaire, sneak Sassy a couple more snacks, and cuddle with Stud until he wriggles free and ponders me from the window ledge.

We need to create genuinely effective methods of calming and containing ourselves so that stress and worry do not interfere with our rest.

To fall asleep, get your body involved in a way that interrupts the agitation in your body. Relaxing in a warm (not hot or cold) bath is helpful for some. Deep breathing exercises can slow us down long enough to fall asleep. Sometimes I get out of bed, lie on my back on the floor (preferably on a rug or padded surface) and, placing a tennis ball underneath the space between my shoulder blades, I "roll" the ball between my shoulder blades by gently moving my back to and fro. This self-massage releases tension I've stored in my back and neck muscles. When I am prompted to take a deep breath or when I enjoy a wide yawn, I know that my body is releasing stress and is preparing to sleep. Experiment to find out what works best for you.

Put Your Face on Your To-Do List

We are goaded into devaluing self-nurturing. We either end up
believing we don't deserve self-care or, if we do, that it must be the
last thing on our mighty list of Things To Do.
—JENNIFER LOUDEN, *The Woman's Comfort Book* (1992)

Is your face feeling neglected? Tired? Ready for some pampering?
Look no further than your refrigerator. Cut up a cucumber (skin
and all) and puree in your blender. Add two tablespoons of plain
yogurt and mix thoroughly. Spread the mixture on your face, being
careful to avoid your eyes. Take the phone off the hook and relax
for half an hour while the mask freshens your skin. The yogurt
contains a natural enzyme that will loosen dead cells and nourish
the new cells emerging. The cucumber acts as an astringent and
will tighten your skin for a healthier glow. Rinse with warm water
and follow with toner.

Listen

Listening is a form of accepting.
—STELLA TERRILL MANN

Our bodies have a wealth of information to share with us, if we will only listen. The non-verbal language of my body may be quite different from yours. For example, a knot in my calf may mean that I've not stood my ground recently and I need to advocate for myself better in the future. A knot in your calf may mean something altogether different, such as fear and the need to flee from a dangerous situation. Someone else may have a knot in her calf because she's been wearing high heels too often! I believe there is no universal decoder ring to decipher what all of our bodies have to say. As Thomas Moore writes in *Care of the Soul,* "There can be no thesaurus of body imagery."

The challenge is to ask your body what a sore muscle or other signal means and then listen. See what idea pops into your head. The more you listen, the better you will get at interpreting your body's language, cooperating and making peace with your body.

Celebrate Your Cycle

When you take a look at nature, you see that the cycles,
whether the winter cycle of hibernation, the lunar cycle of tides, or
the twenty-four-hour circadian cycle of rest and activity,
all have some kind of renewal component that
promotes growth in the particular system they govern.
—NANCY LONSDORF, M.D., VERONICA BUTLER, M.D., AND MELANIE
BROWN, PH.D., *A Woman's Best Medicine* (1995)

I began my period on the second day of seventh grade. Back in those days, we attached pads the size of small mattresses to clamps on elastic belts worn around our waists. I was the same five-feet, six-inches I am today but at least twenty pounds thinner, so keeping those belts on my hips was quite a challenge. The whole idea struck me as comical. As time went on, however, I developed cramps and grew to dread the appearance of blood.

One way we can make peace with our periods is to look at the bigger picture of how our personal cycles are intertwined with the many other cycles in nature. All cycles have death and rebirth aspects, with loss making room for new growth. As Doctors Lonsdorf, Butler, and Brown write, "Once we understand the menstrual cycle as a purifying mechanism for keeping the bodymind prepared for wholeness, we recognize its purpose beyond reproduction as a regular opportunity for eliminating the accumulation of . . . waste products that have the potential to give rise to illness."

How do you view your period? Record in your body journal what your period means to you. Rather than viewing menstruation as a negative experience, contemplate the cleansing aspects of your flow. Share your feelings with your body buddy, expressing gratitude for the cycle within you linking you with the rhythm of nature.

Don't Assume Safety

There is no person who is not dangerous for someone.
—MARIE DE SÉVIGNÉ, *Letters of Madame de Sévigné*
to Her Daughter and Friends (1811)

I've made the painful mistake of trying to divide the world into dangerous and safe people, as if certain individuals are always dangerous and others are always safe. I've gotten into trouble not because I stayed away from those whom I believed to be dangerous, but because I let my guard down around those whom I assumed would or could never harm me.

I'm not talking about cruel people but my closest and dearest loved ones. In fact, I have inflicted pain on myself through disliking my body or depriving myself of what I need. If I can't rely on myself to keep myself perfectly safe, how can I expect that from anyone else?

In graduate school, one of my favorite professors taught us that every good deed has at least one negative, unintended consequence. That idea shattered my simplistic notion that if I intended to do good, good would always result. I've unintentionally hurt others—for example the time I sent flowers to a friend, not realizing she had allergies. And I've unintentionally hurt myself—like the time I sprained my ankle while learning self-defense or the time I gave myself diarrhea by taking too much vitamin C. My intention is good, but I can't completely control all the possible outcomes. None of us can.

We're all dangerous to some extent to ourselves and others, regardless of our desire to contribute positively. Remember that in every good intention lies a risk and that in the heart of everyone who loves us is a shadow no one can control.

Share a Salad

*You can put everything, and the more things the better,
into a salad, as into a conversation; but everything
depends upon the skill of mixing.*
—CHARLES DUDLEY WARNER

In the darkness of late November, create something that reminds you of the spring that will come. Make a fabulous salad with everything you can imagine—different types of lettuce such as curly endive, escarole, chicory, roquette, or watercress. Don't settle for the standard tomato garnish. Be creative with pomegranate seeds, seedless grapes, pepper slices, sliced onion, mint leaves, apple slices, and raisins. (I'm making myself hungry. . . .)

Once you've created your masterpiece, invite someone special to share it with you. Talk about your plans for the next summer. Your body will benefit from both the meal and the conversation.

Examine Your Breasts

Nature has made women with a bosom, so nature thought it was important. Who am I to argue with nature?
—IDA ROSENTHAL, Inventor of the modern brassiere

Over the years, I've discovered two lumps in my breasts. Both times they turned out to be fluid-filled cysts that were drained in a nearly painless office procedure. My experience is common, since most breast lumps turn out to be benign.

Often the fear of cancer causes us women to keep our hands off our breasts. We're afraid of what we'll find. Remember, even if the lump you find turns out to be malignant, breast cancer is curable if, and only if, it is detected early enough to get the treatment needed.

Examine your breasts the same time each month. First stand in front of a mirror and see if you notice any changes in size, shape, or color. Next, lie down and raise one of your arms over your head. Working on the breast on the same side as your raised arm and moving in a circular direction, slowly feel for thickening tissue or lumps. Make sure you examine your entire breast. Examine your nipples and under your arms. Lastly, squeeze your nipple for any discharge. Repeat this process on your other breast.

If you find anything suspicious, call your doctor right away. Don't delay. Chances are your experience will be similar to mine, a bit nerve-racking but of no major concern. And if there is a malignancy, catching it early can make all the difference.

DECEMBER

ALIVE

I want to be screamingly alive,
with birth and growth
and the terrible real of things.

It is terrible to be alive.
To know. To see. To acknowledge.
To grieve forever the loss, the outrage.

But I long to have the courage
and the wonder to bear Life.

I long to be made of sturdy stuff
that can hold the searing pain of being.

I want to hold the pain
without spilling it onto others,
without pretense of bravery,
without frightened retreats
into the thousand deaths that I have historically taken.

I want to hold the pain
not as a martyr but as a mortal,
humbled by the anguish of my limits.

I want to hold the pain
so that it can carve my soul into something real.

I want to hold the pain
until it is time to realize some part of it, transformed
into compassion, quiet joy,
and a raucous laughter at it all.

Prepare for Change

Surely the two mysteries of life are birth and death. These events we can never understand fully. . . . What we can do is tell the story of our birth, of our life, and of the lives and deaths of those we love, what they mean to us and what they meant to us, how they touched us and how they shaped us.
—CAMILLE LITTLETON HEGG, *Women of the Word: Contemporary Sermons by Women Clergy* (1985)

The holiday season confronts us with the complexities of change. The calendar year comes to an end, triggering reflective thoughts like, "Where did the time go?" and "Did I accomplish all I wanted to this year?" and "I've enjoyed this year and hate to see it go." We're reminded of the personal changes we wanted to make in diet, exercise, stress management, and enjoyment. Some of our goals have been achieved, others haven't. Some changes we celebrate, others we still desire.

As the year ends, we also receive the opportunity to start anew. We can set new goals, rely on understanding we didn't have a year ago, and make changes that enhance our lives. We're surrounded by songs and visual images of mother and baby, reminding us women in particular that our bodies are specially created for the birthing process. With or without pregnancy, we can trust our bodies to lead us to rebirth and renewal.

If our bodies teach us anything, it is to expect change. In the years in which we have experienced life as an embodied soul, our bodies have changed in size and shape. As we grew, so did our capabilities, as we learned to walk, talk, and use our hands effectively. We came to depend on our capabilities and were dismayed when these were hampered through illness, accidents, or aging.

Our bodies have also taught us about the predictability and inevitability of death and rebirth. We've all experienced small deaths, or losses, through the diminished functioning, pain, and emotional distress which accompany the illnesses we've suffered. Each time we recover from an illness, our bodies teach us that we are equipped for surviving. In fact, if our pain and sicknesses are seen as invitations for deeper understanding, we can use these experiences for positive change.

Through our bodies new life is brought into this world. And in our bodies we will eventually experience death. I do not believe that death is an ending of our lives but yet another change, a new beginning. I rest my confidence in all God has taught me through my body regarding the cycle of death and rebirth.

Rather than allow change to take you by surprise, prepare for change by learning from the wisdom of your body. Be secure in the predictability of change.

Dance through the Holidays

In our haste to make it to Christmas, we often fill our waiting with frantic steps. We may dance a frenzied tarantella of shopping, baking, Christmas card writing, decorating, and caring for others. We wear ourselves out in the process and then wonder why our spirits sink after the holidays. Or we may dance a slow, painful dance of aloneness, wishing that the images of happy, prosperous families and friends would hurry up and pass for another year.
—JAN L. RICHARDSON, *Sacred Journeys* (1995)

What sort of dance do you intend to dance during this holiday? How will you move your body through the days between now and the new year? Will you over-commit yourself to an excessively busy schedule, running on adrenaline, only to collapse in exhaustion once the decorations are back in the boxes? Or will you slowly drag yourself through the motions, senses muted, missing out on all the tastes, sights, smells, sounds, and sensations of the season?

We all have a choice to make about our holiday dance. Make yours a graceful, grace-filled movement led by the rhythm of your body's need for pleasure and comfort. Jot down a few ways you can lighten your load. Perhaps you should send Fourth of July cards instead of Christmas cards, do your shopping through catalogs (where they do the shipping), or combine baking and socializing with a cookie baking party. Take time for the simple experiences of the senses, stroll rather than rush through the holidays, and listen for the spiritual wisdom available to you in the peacefulness.

Locate Longing in Your Body

It seems to me we can never give up longing and wishing while we are thoroughly alive. There are certain things we feel to be beautiful and good, and we must hunger after them.
—GEORGE ELIOT, *The Mill on the Floss* (1860)

Sometimes longing for someone special to love can feel so visceral that it's hard for me to distinguish between the emotion and the physical sensation. Longing finds its expression through my chest, right between my breasts, as a heaviness that demands my attention. Sometimes causing me to wonder if I'm having a heart attack, longing presses down on me, nearly overpowering me.

How does your body express longing? Where in your body do you feel pangs of wishing and desire? Describe your body's expression in your body journal. This is the first step in responding to your longings and needs. If you feel comfortable, share your longings with your body buddy or someone else you trust.

Celebrate Your Skin

*The skin itself does not think, but its sensitivity is so great, combined
with its ability to pick up and transmit so extraordinarily wide a
variety of signals, and make so wide a range of responses,
exceeding that of all other sense organs, that for versatility
it must be ranked second only to the brain itself.*
—ASHLEY MONTAGU, *Touching* (1986)

Why does touch communicate so powerfully to us?
Soon after conception, as our cells are dividing and
developing, the skin and the central nervous system originate from
the same tissue. Dr. Ashley Montagu, author of *Touching*, writes,
"The nervous system is . . . a buried part of the skin and alternatively
the skin may be regarded as an exposed portion of the nervous
system." When someone touches our skin, they are in essence
touching our nervous system. No wonder we respond so strongly
to all kinds of touch, from friendly handshakes or soft caresses to
painful slaps or bruising blows.

Stroke your skin today in a soothing manner, knowing that you
are not merely stroking the surface of your body but are affecting
your interior nervous system.

Step to the Side

*We are going to do something terrible to you—
we are going to deprive you of an enemy.*
—SOVIET REPRESENTATIVE, addressing the United States at the
dismantling of the Soviet Union

S ome people are not happy unless they have an enemy—a neighbor with whom to argue, a group to distrust and hate, a reason for conflict and heated debate. Know anyone like this? I do. People like this seem to come into my life with an alarming regularity.

I used to try to negotiate with anyone who had some complaint or concern, but I have learned over the years that some people don't want resolution. Some people are happy only when they're angry at someone else. However, we aren't required to take on every challenge that comes our way. Our bodies have only so much energy, and allowing one person to repeatedly trigger the "fight or flight" response can wear one down. How would you rather use that energy? Fighting with someone who refuses to let the conflict resolve?

When trying to work things out won't help, the best defense is not fighting but getting out of the way. Don't engage your body in the fray. Be safe, be wise, and step to the side.

Enjoy a Simple Pleasure

A simple enough pleasure, surely,
to have breakfast alone with one's husband,
but how seldom married people in the midst of life achieve it.
—ANNE MORROW LINDBERGH, *Gift from the Sea* (1955)

How often do you enjoy simple pleasures? As a rule, most of us rush through our lives, rarely slowing down for sensuous experiences. In fact, many of us fear sensuousness, as if by connecting to our bodies and the joys of our senses, we may spiral out into some wild, out-of-control debauchery.

Actually, the most sensuous experiences are often quite safe and usually bring us closer to those we love. We cannot experience the joys of our senses unless we slow down and take time to savor the moment with our loved ones.

Today's exercise is to share a sensuous moment with someone you love—a friend, lover, child, or parent. Share a meal—breakfast, brunch, afternoon tea, or dinner. No need to make a big fuss over the fixings. Make it simple. Share a loaf of fresh bread, cheese, and soup. Perhaps fresh apples, warm muffins, and juice. Or maybe hot tea, scones, and jelly.

Don't rush. Take time to savor the tastes. Slowly digest the nourishing food. Give yourself the time to digest the love you exchange in these sacred and sensual moments of pleasure and intimacy.

Get a Jump on the Holidays

No matter how you choose to move, it should be for the purpose of experiencing and enjoying your body, regardless of your shape. We are entitled to this kind of pleasure.
—JANE R. HIRSCHMANN AND CAROL H. MUNTER,
When Women Stop Hating Their Bodies (1995)

As a kid I used to love the holidays—unwrapping presents, eating favorite foods, seeing relatives I rarely saw otherwise, getting a vacation from school. But as I've grown older, other images have replaced these positive ones, such as feeling financially stressed by the gift-giving, feeling overwhelmed by all there is to accomplish, and remembering family members who have passed away and are no longer around to enjoy the season with me.

Instead of letting the holidays get you down, jump into the new year with enthusiasm. And I do mean this literally! Get a jump rope and take a couple of minutes each day to hop like you did when you were a little girl. I guarantee that it's impossible to jump rope and feel down at the same time! Jumping gets the blood pumping, the endorphins flowing, and the giggles breaking through that "bah humbug"demeanor.

One way or the other, you'll get everything done this year, just like you have every year before this. Only this year, with jump rope in hand, you'll feel younger and experience more of the season's childlike wonder.

Say What You Want

Want, the Mistress of Invention, still tempts me on . . .
—SUSANNA WESLEY, *The Busy Body* (1709)

Visit any mall and you'll see Santa with children in his lap, listening to what they want to receive this Christmas. As children, we were encouraged to put our wants into words and to expect Santa (or someone) to respond. But as we grow older, telling others what we genuinely desire can be more difficult.

Take out your body journal and sit for a moment, checking in with your body. Do you need nourishment—touch, food, play? Is your energy level high or are you worn out? Ask your body to help you identify what you need and want right now. Then reword these items and experiences in your body journal. Give yourself the opportunity to say these desires out loud by sharing your list with your body buddy.

Sing Your Song

*A bird does not sing because it has an answer—
it sings because it has a song.*
—CHINESE PROVERB

Recently I spoke at a conference and, upon leaving the platform, a woman came up to me and said, "You look ten years younger than your picture. I mean, it's a nice picture and all, but get rid of it!"

I laughed out loud, it was such a weird compliment. I remember when I got that set of pictures made. I was feeling down and frustrated with a number of things in my life. I guess it showed. Even though years have passed since that picture was taken, my life continues to improve the more I heed the guidance I get from my body and change things in my life accordingly. While I don't pretend to have it all together, I feel more fulfilled now than at any previous time in my life.

Are you doing what you're meant to be doing? Are you singing your song? Our bodies respond favorably when we're engaged in activities that are fulfilling to us. Bodies seem to age more rapidly when we feel trapped or when we feel like we are wasting our lives. I believe that each of us has a purpose here on earth. Fulfilling that purpose may require that we go against the grain, since we live in a society that values conformity and living up to other people's expectations. Creatively finding our individual paths may frighten or annoy some people. Joy will be your body's confirmation of your choices. The more you insist on being the woman you were meant to be, the more joy you will be blessed with, the way a bird is blessed with a song.

Get Attention

*If you received the blessing of physical kindness and attention from
your parents, these are feelings you wish to return to, and
if you never received such tender nurturance and affection,
this is a state you long to finally arrive at.*
—DAPHNE ROSE KINGMA, *True Love* (1991)

Give me attention!
Ever hear your heart crying out this longing? We all need
attention because we all need love. We know someone cares when
they look us in the eye, touch our hand, listen to us tell our story, or
in some way demonstrate care.

Be clear with yourself today about what kind of attention you
need. Do you need some visual attention? Maybe you need to receive
a smile from a friend, share the view with your partner, or watch a
film all by yourself in the afternoon. Are you in need of auditory
affirmation? Give a friend a call just to hear her voice or ask a co-
worker to share lunch with you so you can chat together. If you're
needing kinesthetic attention, you might ask for a hug or share a
sensual massage with your partner. Let your body receive the
attention you need.

Celebrate Selfishness

*Creative selfishness, like all self-nurturing activities, will help you
amass an overflow of love that will allow you
to care for others from your abundance.*
—JENNIFER LOUDEN, *The Woman's Comfort Book* (1992)

B usy taking care of everyone else but yourself? Holiday
preparations beginning to take more and more of your time?

Take a break and cultivate some selfishness. Use your imagination
and take yourself to someplace warm. Play some calypso music to
set the mood. Take two bananas and mash one in a bowl. Stir in a
teaspoon of honey and a dash of cream. Once you have mixed it
thoroughly, gently smooth this delicious mixture on your face, being
careful to avoid your eyes.

Lose yourself in the music. While you are relaxing, the banana
will draw out impurities, and the honey and cream will nourish
your skin. Let the mask do all the work. Slowly peel the second
banana and munch slowly, giving your mouth a tropical taste treat.
After a few minutes, remove the mask with warm water and follow
with a toner.

Wouldn't you agree that selfishness has gotten an unnecessarily
bad name?

Assess Your Stress

Always do one thing less than you can do.
—BERNARD BARUCH

The other day I told a friend that my new year's resolution was to be bored. Somehow sitting around, feeling like there's nothing pressing to do sounds absolutely delicious to me right now! While I don't really want to feel disinterested in life, I believe my desire for boredom serves as an indicator that there's too much stress and not enough satisfying challenges in my life.

How about you? What does your body tell you about the stress in your life? Time to bring out your body journal and draw an outline of your body. Mark in the areas of your body that are telling you there are too many unfulfilling demands in your life. Notice the tension headache, the lower back pain, the bladder infection. Pay attention to the overeating, the nervousness, the inability to focus attention. These are helpful signs that changes need to be made.

Share

Sharing is sometimes more demanding than giving.
—MARY CATHERINE BATESON, *Composing a Life* (1989)

In 1985 I suffered a colossal burnout after trying to take care of others while pretending I had no needs of my own. Of course to attempt such a feat, I also had to pretend I had no body. Perched on my pedestal, giving dutifully to others, I thought I was safe from harm. But believe me, falling (or should I say collapsing) off that pedestal was painful, forcing me to confront my own needs and my body. During the past decade, I've learned there's a big difference between giving to someone and sharing with someone.

We can give to others without being vulnerable or sharing anything intimate about ourselves. Sharing implies a level of vulnerability inherent in mutuality. As givers, we can take on a superior, even impersonal position in the interaction. As sharers, we too become vulnerable, revealing our own needs and wounds. And vulnerability implies permeability. When we are open to others, we can take in affection and love as well as give it.

Take time today to share with another woman whom you trust to be mutually vulnerable. Share with each other where you are in the process of making peace with your bodies. Resist the urge to give advice. Come down from the pedestal and enjoy the rich intimacy and support possible only between two equals. The joy of sharing is well worth the risks.

Sweep Out Your Stomach

Spinach is the broom of the stomach.
—FRENCH PROVERB

Ah, roughage. Don't we hear a lot about the need to eat whole grains, fresh fruits, and vegetables and to drink freshly squeezed juices? Today, let's clean house by tossing this interior cleanser into your juicer:

♦ A handful of spinach
♦ 4-5 carrots, greens removed
♦ 2 small apples
♦ 2 stalks of celery

I'll admit it doesn't taste quite as good as a root beer float, but it is drinkable and sooo healthy!

Be Still

Happiness lies in the fulfillment of the spirit through the body.
—CYRIL CONNOLLY (1903-1974)

You're halfway through the month and probably inundated with holiday preparations and shopping. Cynthia Bohnker writes in her helpful guide, *Overcoming Holiday Stress,* "The 'perfect' Christmas, with all the trimmings, all the invitations to events, close relationships with family and friends—just the thought of orchestrating it can be both exhausting and overwhelming."

Take a few moments today and remove yourself from all the hubbub. When arriving at your next appointment or errand, turn the car off and sit for a couple of minutes (or until your car gets cold). Relax into the quietness of your body. Take several deep breaths, letting go of holiday stress with each exhale. Breathe in spiritual renewal with each inhale. Remind yourself of God's presence and the comfort available to you any time of day. Even in the middle of the busiest time of year.

Relax!

How beautiful it is to do nothing, and then rest afterward.
—SPANISH PROVERB

The Puritans never heard this proverb. Those of us who have been influenced by values extolling the virtues of hard work, self-denial, and busyness need to meditate on this one. Your assignment today is to carve out some time in which nothing whatsoever of importance is accomplished.

Enjoy a do-nothing day (or at least a do-nothing evening). Let the stress flow from your body as you put together a jigsaw puzzle, watch a video, or concentrate on your breath for twenty minutes or so.

And then, after all this exertion, take a nap.

Make Amends with Your Body

Negative self-esteem . . . is a form of emotional self-abuse.
When the core of the self is vulnerable to attack,
we are often our own worst enemy.
—RAY S. ANDERSON, *Self Care* (1995)

Since the third grade, I've never looked someone in the eye and yelled, "You are stupid and ugly!" (I was quite verbal in my youth.) Calling someone names like this is no longer in my repertoire—that is, unless that someone is me.

When I am the target of my wrath, I am quite apt to use such words as idiot, useless, ugly, yucky, awful, weak, and bad. I can say cruel things to my body without any awareness of how damaging such self-talk can be.

Are you your own worst enemy? Perhaps today is the day to apologize, the same way you would if you verbally abused a friend. Take steps to make amends. Your body does not deserve your cruelty, just your acceptance and your love.

Celebrate Movement

I finally discovered the source of all movement,
the unity from which all diversities of movement are born.
—ISADORA DUNCAN (1877-1927)

From time to time, I close my shutters for privacy and put a drumming tape into the player. With the wild beats pulsating through my body, I'll stomp, swing, flail, and shuffle to my heart's content. No one watching. No one judging. No specific steps to master, just me and my body out to have a great time. When the tape ends, I'm happy and my body's happy. It's amazing, but I always feel at peace with my body after a drum dance.

Take time to move today. Depending on what your local weather is like, here are some ideas:

♦ Hike up a mountain trail.
♦ Grab a partner for a night of country western dancing.
♦ Climb on a jungle gym at a local park.
♦ Play a rigorous game of racquetball.
♦ Slam balls at a neighborhood batting center.
♦ Glide over the ice at the community rink.
♦ Start a beginner's ballet class.
♦ Jump rope.
♦ Swim several laps across the pool.
♦ Put on fifties music and do the twist.

Lots of ways to move!

Keep Your Eyes Open

Watch out, my dear,
there's a scorpion under every stone.
—PRAXILLA, untitled fragment, 451 B.C.

While some of us are thinking about what we can give to others this holiday season, some unsavory characters are plotting to take whatever they can from others. With all the shopping going on, thieves are all the more intent on robbing holiday shoppers, so be alert and keep your eyes open.

Pay heightened attention to the moments during shopping that you are especially vulnerable, such as when you are leaving a store, walking to your car, putting packages in your car, or driving home. If possible, shop with a friend or family member so that you can have an extra pair of eyes watching for anyone who might be watching you. Ever since I was held up, I carry a portable phone with me in case I need to call 911 immediately.

Be alert and keep your eyes open. You'll make a less desirable target.

Prepare for Age Regression

Do you become an eight-year-old when you're with your growing-up family, when you're really 28, 38, 48, 58 or 68? Does it feel like they treat you the same way you experienced as a kid?
—CYNTHIA BOHNKER, *Overcoming Holiday Stress* (1995)

Who hasn't felt that weird transformation from competent adult to bumbling child while walking up to the door of a family member? You got out of the car with all your capabilities, confident of your accomplishments, but by the time the door opened, there you were feeling small and vulnerable. As holiday family gatherings threaten to beam you back into your childhood, here are three things you can do when the family heat is on:

Bring a friend: Keeping contact with someone who knows us as we are now can keep us in the present. If you're married, having your spouse with you is helpful. If not, invite a friend along. Take small breaks to check in with your "people" to remind you that yes, you are actually an adult and not a little girl.

Remember to breathe: Some of my clients stop breathing at the mention of certain family members. If your family situation is stressful, expect that at important times, especially challenging moments, you'll hold your breath. This is a natural reaction to danger. However, holding your breath opens the door to losing contact with the present. Check in periodically to see if you are breathing. Take several deep breaths, reminding yourself that you're an adult.

Anchor yourself: Select a body part that will serve as an anchor to adulthood. One woman I know walks barefoot on the carpet to ground herself. I touch my fingers together. Experiment with what will work for you, such as running cold water over your hands, biting an apple, or looking in the mirror.

Develop a Taste for Healthy Food

Fake food—I mean those patented substances chemically flavored
and mechanically bulked out to kill the appetite
and deceive the gut—is unnatural, almost immoral,
a bane to good eating and good cooking.
—JULIA CHILD, *Julia Child and Company* (1978)

Every Christmas a small group of friends comes over to my place for our annual "Tacky Christmas Party." We compete for who can bring the tackiest gift and who can wear the tackiest Christmas outfit. And we share a potluck of tacky food.

Excitedly, we munch on all-meat wieners, wrapped in white bread (now I just eat the bread); processed cheese out of a can onto greasy potato chips; and dessert on powdered-sugar doughnuts. Basically, we eat the processed food we all ate as kids. Then these items were cool. Now, they are kind of disgusting. They're also not very nutritious, if not downright detrimental to health.

Developing a taste for fresh food has not been easy for me. I'm still not the first in line for the high-fiber, low-fat recipes. But I am getting better at enjoying the two to four servings of fruit we're all supposed to be eating every day. How are you doing in this department? Have you had a luscious orange, a sweet pear, or a slice of apple today? I'll try to eat right, if you will.

But I must admit, I still look forward to that one party a year, when I get to eat all those awful, tacky, processed foods. Too bad fat, salt, and sugar aren't considered food groups!

Celebrate Your Body

If I had influence with the good fairy who is supposed to preside over the christening of all children I should ask that her gift . . . be a sense of wonder so indestructible that it would last throughout life.
—RACHEL CARSON, *The Sense of Wonder* (1965)

Write in the numbers indicating how often, if ever, the statements are true. Modify those statements that don't apply to you. 1—Never, 2—Sometimes, 3—Always.

___I celebrate my body by getting proper rest.

___I celebrate my body by eating nutritious food.

___I celebrate my body by keeping my weight at a healthy level.

___I celebrate my body by exercising regularly.

___I celebrate my body by breathing deeply and calmly.

___I celebrate my body by wearing comfortable clothing.

___I celebrate my feet by wearing good shoes.

___I celebrate my skin with proper cleaning and moisturizing.

___I celebrate my back by standing correctly.

___I celebrate my breasts by regular self-exams.

___I celebrate my breasts by wearing beautiful bras.

___I celebrate my genitals through proper hygiene.

___I do not tolerate pain.

___My friends often compliment my body.

___I regularly receive massage as a way to celebrate my body.

Scoring Evaluation

37-45   Congratulations! You have a high regard for your body.
26-36   Watch out. Your body-attitude needs improvement.
0-25   Body alert! Your body deserves a lot more attention.

Heed the Message

If you don't heed the message the first time,
you get hit with a bigger hammer the next time.
—CHRISTIANE NORTHRUP, M.D., *Women's Bodies,*
Women's Wisdom (1994)

A young boy called, "Mom, look at me!" gleefully wearing the hat the pilot loaned him, wanting his mother to share his joy. I watched him tug at his mother's sleeve as we were boarding the plane. Focused on getting the tickets ready for the flight attendant, she ignored her son's attempts to get her attention. But he would not be dissuaded. He called her name and tugged even harder. Again she ignored him. Finally in frustration he pinched her arm. "Ow!" she yelped, snapping in his direction. "Why in the world did you do that?" she asked angrily.

I knew exactly why he had pinched her. He'd tried repeatedly in more subtle, less painful ways to get her attention. But she had ignored him. Not until he had caused her pain, and a sufficient amount, did she look up and notice something was amiss.

Most of us treat our bodies like this mother did her son. At first, our bodies give us small messages such as a twitching eyelid or an upset stomach. If we ignore the signs, the body turns up the volume on the pain indicator. Our eye becomes infected or we throw up our lunch. If we still miss the point, and often we do, our bodies will become even more demonstrative. The infection spreads into our throat or we develop diarrhea along with the vomiting. Pay attention to the little pain messages your body is sending. You may avoid getting hit over the head.

Look at Your Body through Eyes of Love

Some of us are so hooked into shame that we are afraid we would be
lonely without it. . . . If we lost our shame,
we would not recognize ourselves.
—LEWIS B. SMEDES, Theologian

What would I look like if I were proud of my body?

I try to envision myself, my body shame-free. Would my spine have grown straighter if I hadn't slouched to hide my embarrassment over being a gangly, uncoordinated ten-year-old unaccustomed to a body five-feet, six-inches tall? Would my skin be smoother and healthier now if as a teenager I hadn't wanted to look like the girls in the magazine ads and repeatedly burned my fair skin in a futile effort to achieve that coveted tan? Would my smile be different if I didn't wear caps to cover the teeth I broke at night, fretfully grinding my teeth in my sleep? How would I breathe, stand, or move if I weren't self-conscious or unsure or fearful?

Let's pretend, just for a moment, with no one else watching, that you and I are thrilled to be who we are. We love ourselves, especially our bodies. Take a moment and stand in front of a full-length mirror. Close your eyes and breathe. Deeply. Take in a sense of well-being. With the exhale, let go of all the shame, the criticisms, the shoulds. Let your body rearrange itself, feeling proud, free, strong, and loved. After as many breaths as it takes to let go of the shame and let your body reacclimate, open your eyes. How do you look now?

Taste Grace

God is spreading grace around in the world like a five-year-old spreads peanut butter; thickly, sloppily, eagerly, and if we are in the back shed trying to stay clean, we won't even get a taste.
—DONNA SCHAPER, *Stripping Down* (1991)

Christmas Day is usually filled with scrumptious things to eat— most of them sweet such as cookies, fudge, and fruitcake. As your mouth enjoys the treats of the holiday, remember that the Christian message is uniquely sweet: Motivated by love for us, God becomes a human being, becomes flesh and blood, just like you and me. Our bodies are not evil encasements or impulses that require taming but are an integral part of the expression of love on all levels— spiritually, physically, and emotionally.

Savor this delicious spiritual truth this Christmas Day. Allow your body to enjoy every sensual experience available. Delight in the smell of crackling oak burning in the fireplace, the twinkle of joy seen in the eyes of children, the melodies of hope wafting through your home. Taste, touch, observe, smell, and listen to the signs of grace all around you. Celebrate the miracle of birth by allowing God's message of embodied grace to permeate every cell in your body.

Beat the Backlash

*All changes, even the most longed for, have their melancholy, for
what we leave behind us is a part of ourselves. We must die to one
life before we can enter another.*
—ANATOLE FRANCE (1844-1924)

The big day has come and gone. The presents are opened, the
wrappings tossed in the trash, the relatives on their way home.
Was Christmas what you hoped for this year?

Check in with your body before you get too far into your day to
discover how you're feeling. Often feelings that were triggered during
Christmas festivities but delayed because of all the excitement come
rushing into our bodies the day after. Knowing your body as you
do, you're prepared to identify and express your feelings more
expertly than you could last year at this time.

Is that anger between your shoulder blades? Regret caught in
your throat? Relief in your abdomen? Weariness in your lower back?
Leftover wishes stuck in your chest? Record these feelings in your
body journal. Check in with your body buddy to see how she fared
this season. Time to acknowledge the triumphs and grieve the losses
of another year. Recognition is the first step to change.

Fan the Light in Others

Start with little things seen through the magnifying glass of wonder,
and just as a magnifying glass can focus the sunlight into a burning
beam that can set a leaf aflame, so can your focused wonder set you
ablaze with insight. Find the light in each other and just fan it.
—ALICE O. HOWELL, *The Dove in the Stone* (1988)

God created each of us with unique talents and gifts. Today, open your eyes to the light in others. Select a woman in your life (maybe your body buddy?) and notice how she brings light into your world. What are the physical components of that gift? Perhaps her smile reminds you that love is real and tangible. Maybe she has a gift of touch, always ready to give your tense shoulder muscles a nurturing squeeze. Perhaps the sound of her voice soothes you when adrenaline is coursing through your veins.

Let her know today how much you appreciate her contribution to your life. You will fan her flame by acknowledging her gifts.

Get and Stay Healthy

Since Everywoman's problem occurs in part because of the nature of being female in this culture, which programs us to put the needs of others ahead of our own, we need to make radical changes in our minds and lives to get and stay healthy.
—CHRISTIANE NORTHRUP, M.D., *Women's Bodies, Women's Wisdom* (1994)

As you look forward to a new year, assess your health habits. Are you making regular decisions that will support your body's natural efforts toward a long and active life? Are you valuing yourself enough to eat more fruits and vegetables, while passing on the processed sugars, salt, and fat? Do you honor your heart and circulatory system by engaging in regular aerobic exercise that you actually enjoy? Are you turning your stressors into challenges, thereby minimizing the damage frustration can have on every cell in your body?

Take stock of how the demands of being a woman, with the various roles we're expected to play, may undermine your health. Set out specific, yet reachable goals that will become next year's health habits. You're worth the effort.

Be Grateful

Is not sight a jewel? Is not hearing a treasure? Is not speech a glory?
O my Lord, pardon my ingratitude and pity my dullness
who am not sensible of these gifts.
—THOMAS TRAHERNE

At moments it seems hard for me to imagine not being madly in love with my body! The delight of feeling a hug from someone I love, hearing the laughter of children, watching my cats romp and play, tasting the sweetness of a kiss. Pausing a moment to recognize the marvel of my heart beating without my having to make it so. Knowing that, as I write, cells within my bloodstream are racing to points of bacterial attack to protect me from illnesses I never knew had invaded my body. My breakfast digests, my lungs fill with air, my cells are nourished while I attend to other details. My feet ground me in a spiritual and physical foundation of confidence and renewal.

What a glorious experience it is to be in one's body. Take time to be grateful for your body. Speak directly to your body, identifying all the ways you appreciate yourself. And then thank the God who created you.

Yearn for Wholeness

We must let our hearts dance and rejoice with love and compassion
and yearn wholeheartedly for oneness and for wholeness.
—CHRISTINA FELDMAN

When I think back on my life before I began to receive body work and massage, I hardly recognize myself. Overwhelmed with oppressive, unruly emotions, I knew that something was very wrong. But I could not comprehend what the problem might be. I didn't know where to start. I couldn't find solid ground. Looking back, I can see why I was unable to make contact with a strong foundation. I was disconnected from my own body. If I was unable to feel my own feet, how could I expect to feel the ground underneath them?

Over the past decade, I've inhabited my body a little bit more each day. As my spirit is reconciled with my body, my emotions reconciled with my intellect and my dreams reconciled with the light of day, joy results. Not that joy has been my goal. It has not been. Wholeness has been my aim. Healing has been the vehicle. But joy, sweet joy, has been my reward.

Take heart if you are discouraged. Continue to yearn for wholeness. Open yourself up to the pain of healing all the various parts of you that may at this moment be at war. Reconciliation is possible, if not inevitable. And when there is wholeness, you'll be immersed in joy.

Accept Your "Good-Enough" Body

When we like ourselves, warts and all, we dance instead of standing around. We walk proud and free instead of shuffling along slump-shouldered. We glow with confidence.
—CARL KOCH AND JOYCE HEIL, *Created in God's Image* (1991)

Researchers are finding out that a parent does not have to be perfect in order to have well-adjusted children. All a mom or dad needs to do is be good enough at paying attention to their children and caring for their needs.

I like this idea when I think about my body. I suppose it's time to let you in on a little secret, just between the two of us—I do not have a perfect body. I'll bet that comes as a shock to you and may cause you to dislike me, but I have to admit it. It isn't perfect. I'm in my forties, and as Gypsy Rose Lee, who paraded her wares publicly, once said, "I have everything I had twenty years ago, only it's a little bit lower." All parts are accounted for, only in a bit different location.

However, my body is good enough. The more I love my good-enough body, the better I feel, the straighter I walk, the more my feet dance, the broader I smile, and the more beautiful I become. For me, good enough is good enough.

Subject Index

Joy

January 1, 8, 15, 22, 29
February 5, 12, 19, 26
March 4, 11, 18, 25
April 8, 10, 22, 29
May 6, 13, 20, 27
June 4, 8, 10, 17, 24
July 1, 8, 15, 22, 29
August 5, 12, 19, 26
September 2, 9, 24
October 7, 14, 21, 28
November 4, 18, 25
December 2, 9, 16, 29

Safety

January 4, 11, 18, 25
February 1, 8, 15, 22, 29
March 7, 14, 21, 28
April 1, 4, 11, 15, 18, 25
May 2, 9, 16, 23, 30
June 3, 6, 13, 20, 27
July 4, 11, 18, 25
August 1, 8, 15, 22, 29
September 5, 12, 19, 26
October 3, 10, 17, 24, 31
November 7, 14, 21, 28
December 5, 12, 19, 26

Wholeness

January 7, 14, 21, 28
February 4, 11, 18, 25
March 3, 10, 17, 24, 31
April 7, 14, 21, 28
May 5, 12, 19, 26
June 2, 16, 23, 30
July 7, 14, 21, 28
August 4, 11, 18, 20, 25
September 1, 8, 15, 17, 22, 29
October 6, 13, 20, 27
November 3, 8, 10, 17
December 1, 8, 15, 23, 30

Suggestions for Further Reading

The publisher and author gratefully acknowledge the sources listed below for various quotations and references used throughout the text.

Bohnker, Cynthia. *Overcoming Holiday Stress: Daily Encouragements for the Christian in Recovery* (Santa Rosa, CA: Vision Books International, 1995).

Calbom, Cherie and Keane, Maureen. *Juicing for Life* (New York: Avery Publishing Group, 1992).

Cameron, Julie. *The Artist's Way* (New York: Tarcher/Putnam, 1992).

Capacchione, Lucia. *Lighten Up Your Body—Lighten Up Your Life* (North Hollywood: Newcastle Publishing Company, 1990).

Chopra, Deepak. *Ageless Body, Timeless Mind* (New York: Harmony Books, 1993).

Juhan, Deane. *Job's Body: A Handbook for Bodywork* (Barrytown, NY: Station Hill Press, 1987).

Kingma, Daphne Rose. *True Love: How to Make Your Relationship Sweeter, Deeper and More Passionate* (Berkeley, CA: Conari Press, 1991).

Koch, Carl and Heil, Joyce. *Created in God's Image* (Winona, MN: Saint Mary's Press, 1991).

Louden, Jennifer. *The Woman's Comfort Book* (San Francisco: HarperCollins, 1992).

Lowen, Alexander. *The Spirituality of the Body* (New York: McMillan Publishing Company, 1990).

Lyn, Judy. *The Sun Always Rises* (Wickenburg, AZ: H.M. Printing, 1990).

Milkman, Harvey and Sunderwirth, Stanley. *Pathways to Pleasure* (New York: HarperCollins, 1986).

Montagu, Ashley. *Touching: The Human Significance of Skin* (New York: HarperCollins, 1986).

Moore, Thomas. *Care of the Soul* (New York: HarperCollins, 1992).

Nelson, James B. *Embodiment: An Approach to Sexuality and Christian Theology* (Minneapolis, MN: Augsburg, 1978).

Northrup, Christiane. *Women's Bodies, Women's Wisdom* (New York: Bantam Books, 1995).

Older, Jules. *Touching is Healing* (New York: Stein and Day, 1982).

Powell, Don R. *365 Health Hints* (New York: Simon & Schuster, 1990).

Quigley, Paxton. *Not An Easy Target* (New York: Simon & Schuster, 1995).

Stoddard, Alexandra. *Daring to Be Yourself* (New York: Avon Books, 1990).

Timms, Robert and Connors, Patrick. *Embodying Healing: Integrating Bodywork and Psychotherapy in Recovery from Childhood Sexual Abuse* (Orwell, VT: Safer Society Press, 1992).

Wells, Carol G. *Right-Brain Sex: How to Reach the Heights of Sensual Pleasure by Releasing the Erotic Power of Your Mind* (New York: Avon Books, 1989).

About the Author

Carmen Renee Berry, M.S.W., M.A., noted author and speaker, is a nationally certified body worker, social worker, and former psychotherapist who instructs people of all ages on how to integrate the body into the journey toward wholeness. Her previous books include *When Helping You is Hurting Me*, *Who's to Blame?*, and *Your Body Never Lies*. Ms. Berry is a graduate of the University of Southern California's School of Social Work and has an M.A. in Social Sciences from Northern Arizona University. She resides in Pasadena, California.

PageMill Press publishes books in the field of psychology and personal growth. Our publications are intended to intellectually challenge and spiritually enlighten the reader to self-reflection, growing consciousness, and the integration of body, soul and mind. The focus of our books is on the mind/body connection, the power of story and myth in illuminating the dynamics of our psyche and culture, the use of dreams in the movement toward wholeness, the role of the unconscious in human interactions, an increased awareness of the body in all of life's activities, and the universal desire for authentic spiritual experience.

For a catalog of our publications or editorial submissions, please write:

PageMill Press
2716 Ninth Street
Berkeley, CA 94710
Phone: (510) 848-3600
Fax: (510) 848-1326
E-mail: Circulus@aol.com